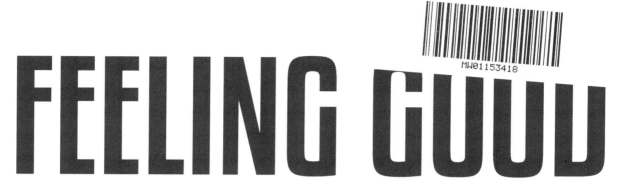

FEELING GOOD

LIVING LOW TOXIN IN COMMUNITY AND EVERYDAY LIFE

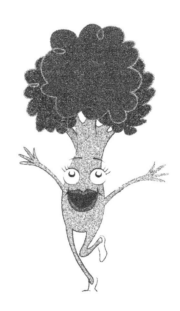

CHERYL MEYER

ILLUSTRATIONS BY NICHOLAS PATTON AND GIZZY DIZZY
EDITED BY JOHN GINS

For permission requests, email the publisher or author at
heavenlytreepress@gmail.com
or send your request to
Heavenly Tree Press
624 E. Winnie Way
Arcadia, CA. 91006

To contact the publisher
heavenlytreepress@gmail.com

To contact the author,
cherylmhealthmuse@gmail.com
ISBN-13: 978-1-7343859-2-2 (Custom Universal)

Library of Congress Control Number:
2020908114

Printed in the United States of America

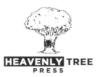

HEAVENLY TREE
PRESS

For more information, contact heavenlytreepress@gmail.com

Disclaimer

The content of this book is for general informational purposes only. It is not meant to be used, nor should it be used to diagnose or treat any medical condition or to replace the services of your physician or other healthcare providers. The advice and strategies contained in the book may not be suitable for all readers. Please consult your healthcare provider for any questions that you may have about your own medical situation. Neither the author, publisher, IIN nor any of their employees or representatives guarantee the accuracy of the information in this book or its usefulness to a particular reader, nor are they responsible for any damage or negative consequence that may result from any treatment, action taken, or inaction by any person reading or following the information in this book.

Heavenly Tree Press

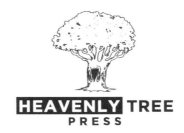

Books by Cheryl Meyer

It Feels Good to Feel Good, Learn to Eliminate Toxins, Reduce Inflammation and Feel Great Again (2017)

It Feels Good to Feel Good, Daily Victory Journal (2019)

It Feels Good to Feel Good, Learn to Eliminate Toxins, Reduce Inflammation and Feel Great Again Second Edition (2020)

Feeling Good: Living Low Toxin in Community and Everyday Life (2020)

Stress—Why Stress is Dangerous to Our Health. Mini Exercises to Do Throughout the Day to Release It. Due (2020)

It Feels Good to Eat the Rainbow—Recipes to Feel Great, Due (2020)

Videos by Cheryl Meyer

Future Proof Your Health—TV Shows are made in cooperation with KGEM, Monrovia, CA. (2020)

Produced by John Gins.
Filmed by Chris Luiten, Operations Manager at KGEM-TV.
Special thank you to David Palomares, Executive Director at KGEM-TV, for all his support to make this a reality.

Future Proof Your Health Videos (2020)

Episode 1: The Benefits of Practicing Gratitude
Episode 2: The Importance of Releasing Stress
Episode 3: Conventional vs. GMO vs. Organic
Episode 4: You are What you Eat
Episode 5: Eat the Rainbow
Episode 6: Get to Know your Farmer's Market
Episode 7: 30 Ways to Save on Healthy Food
Episode 8: Turn Any Recipe Healthy
Episode 9: Eating Healthy Out in Restaurants
Episode 10: The Wonders of Trees

For more information https://heavenlytreepress.com
Https://cherylmhealthmuse.com
Cheryl is available for one on one health coaching.

Cheryl is also available for corporate speaking.

Top subjects that she speaks on:

- It Feels Good to Feel Good—Future Proof Your Health—12 things to start doing today.
- Food Quality Matters—Breaking the Confusion About Food. What SHOULD You Be Eating for Your Health and Your Family's Health?
- If Only I Had Wonder Woman's Superpowers—Fighting Dr. Poison and the Duke of Deception (Where are the poisons and toxins in your life? What can you replace them with?)
- Lose Weight Without Dieting—Count Toxic Chemicals, Not Calories, and Learn the Keys to Unlock Weight Loss.
- Toxic Stress—Simple Exercises to Significantly Reduce it and improve productivity.

You can contact Cheryl at cherylmhealthmuse@gmail.com

Or at 626 399-2304

Dedication

This book is dedicated to people with pain, inflammation, and chronic illness. It is also dedicated to people who want to raise healthy families and are unaware of all the toxins in our world and that lowering toxic load can help their children heal.

It is dedicated to all the people struggling with any of the 100+ autoimmune diseases, cancer, strokes, heart disease, Alzheimer's, Parkinson's, depression, autism, type I and type II diabetes, obesity, psoriasis, eczema, asthma, and hay fever. It is dedicated to children struggling with type I or II diabetes, obesity, ADHD, skin diseases, seizures, autism, and asthma. These people have reached their toxic load and have toppled over the top into chronic illness.

It is also dedicated to all the people who are well but don't want to topple into toxic load, and who want to grow old with dignity and cognizance.

A special thank you to Shilpa Sayana, MD, for encouraging me to write this book for others suffering from chronic illness.

A special thank you to Lea Woodford, my book coach, for her wise encouragement and expertise to get this book completed and to be this comprehensive.

And finally thank you to my husband, John Gins, for his diligence in editing this book, and allowing it to be in my voice. His attention to detail and his ability to be my grammar and spelling police are appreciated beyond words. He is my true partner in crime and my soul mate.

Table of Contents

Foreword

Until it happens, no one is truly prepared for debilitating autoimmune disease or any chronic illness. My friend Cheryl Meyer decided to take her health into her own hands, and research healthier alternatives to autoimmune disease after traditional medical treatments repeatedly failed her and worsened her condition. She has not only healed herself but has become an advocate for those who want to experience better health with more natural alternatives. She skillfully navigates a more natural lifestyle program in this book.

This book is an encyclopedia of natural remedies and healthcare for those wishing to take a more proactive approach to their health. If you or someone you love is suffering from autoimmune disease, cancer, or heart disease, then this book is a must-read. Her book is an easy read and common-sense approach. The book is thoroughly researched, and sources credited accordingly.

Cheryl also addresses children and pets in this book. It is a comprehensive guide to healing yourself and those you love. I highly recommend keeping **It Feels Good to Feel Good, Learn to Eliminate Toxins, Reduce Inflammation and Feel Great Again**, Cheryl's first book close at hand as your go-to guide and resource for healthier alternatives. **Feeling Good, Living in Community in Everyday Life** guides you to maintaining your health with your next steps in an unhealthy world.

Lea Woodford, CEO SmartFem Media Group

Preface

My life today is different from when I woke up eight years ago in horrific pain with autoimmune disease. My life is so different now that it's hard to recognize me as the same woman. And other than getting ill, the changes have all been good!

I sometimes joke that one of the best things to happen to me in my life was that I got autoimmune disease.

Don't get me wrong. If I had a do-over, I would have learned all the things I have learned since that moment, BEFORE I got sick. I would have learned them in time so that I would have avoided all the pain that I went through and have now gotten past, and before my autoimmune disease was irreversible.

Although I no longer have pain, I will always have autoimmune disease.

But getting sick certainly caught my attention. It was the 2x4 hitting my head that I couldn't ignore. My toxic load toppled over the top; I had to react.

I broke up from a long-term toxic relationship; I found another that was perfect for me, and he is my true partner. I married him five years ago.

I have guested on over 100 podcasts, and I have discovered I love sharing my story and helping others.

I sold my jewelry business and have jumped "all in" to share what I learned about health with others that need the information.

I published my first book **It Feels Good to Feel Good, Learn to Eliminate Toxins, Reduce Inflammation and Feel Great Again**, and it has won 13 awards. A new updated version has just been published on Amazon.

I have spoken in 15 summits to share my story and information, and I am scheduled to do two more.

I have started my local community access TV show called **It Feels Good to Feel Good, Futureproof Your Health**. It will debut in March 2020 in my immediate community. This show will then become a podcast in mid-2020 on RHG TV/Voice America, and I will also be including interviews with others who got sick, made lifestyle changes, and returned to relative wellness.

I have started my private Facebook group of the same name as this book, **Feeling Good Living Low Toxin**. The group has people with chronic illnesses looking for solutions to ease their pain, Moms who have sick children, pregnant women who want to birth healthy children, women who want to do all the right things before getting pregnant, and also health coaches who want to learn more about toxins and how they are impacting their clients health.

My goal is to give hope to others with chronic illness and to moms raising children. Changing their lifestyle can make a significant improvement in their health. It is also to help well people stay well before their toxic load topples over the top into illness. My total goal is to impart knowledge to everyone so that they do NOT follow my path to illness. I want to reach others BEFORE they get sick.

I didn't plan on any of this when I got sick. None of this would have happened if I were still well.

It's been a long journey back to the light.

It started with a conventional MD running tests and then running more and yet more and finally calling me to tell me:

1. Nothing was wrong with me.
2. She was going to prescribe steroids to me.

3. I needed to seek mental therapy if I wanted to be pain-free; otherwise, I would be on the steroids for the rest of my life.

Hunh? Why would I take steroids if I had a mental condition?

I knew I hurt. My pain was the worse I had ever experienced. Every joint and every muscle in my body hurt. So, I KNEW something was wrong with me.

And why would I take steroids if nothing was wrong? Unfortunately, I hear similar stories all the time from others who are seeking help from conventional medicine, and their doctors are throwing pills at them or dismissing their symptoms.

I just read a comment from a functional MD that the best thing that could happen to conventional medicine is if all the conventional MD's got a serious illness. They would have to figure out how to help themselves. This is how most functional MDs became "functional." They got sick and looked for a better way to get themselves back to health.

I just read a statistic that most oncologists would not follow their own protocol if they got cancer. (This, of course, depends upon the type of cancer.) Conventional medicine is broken, but there are holistic approaches we can each take to support our own bodies.

At the time I got sick, I owned my own jewelry business and had a well-trained loyal staff, so I turned my business over to them and dug into the research to figure out what was wrong with me.

I didn't even know what I was looking for.

The net result was that I figured out I had an autoimmune disease (the diagnosis was verified by a functional doctor a year later.) I researched and discovered many of the keys to my health. The functional MD I found looked at my body from a different perspective than my conventional MD, and immediately started looking for the root causes of my disease.

I discovered there were two things I could do for myself, and these are the same things that you can do for your own health whether you are well, or you are sick.

I could lower my stress, and I could eliminate toxins. I found ways to lower my stress, and I shared the early things that I learned to reset my parasympathetic nervous system in my first book. It's so important, I have shared it again in this book. My cortisol was so low by the time I got to my Functional MD. I was almost to Addison's disease. She recommended easy ways for me to rebuild my DHEA and to lower my chronic fatigue. Under her guidance, Shilpa Sayana, MD lead me back to relative wellness.

I then dug into where the toxins were. What were they, where could I research, and what would I replace them with? In the end, I eliminated hundreds of toxins from my life. And, this was the significant part, I replaced them all with low toxin items. If you choose to follow my path, each toxin eliminated is a step back towards health. Health can happen, but you need to commit to not follow our American lifestyle and diet.

I shared all this in my book, **It Feels Good to Feel Good, Learn to Eliminate Toxins, Reduce Inflammation and Feel Great Again**, which is the manual that I wish I had when I got ill. In the back of my book, I list all the Functional MD's that I now follow and continue to learn from. It's a great list of references for you to utilize.

I wrote my first book to help others who found themselves in my situation, without hope, frustrated and very sick, and not knowing where to turn. I have met so many people like me. So, I returned to school at 67 and became a health coach so that I could help others. I am now 71, and I am feeling better than I did at 50.

Like others with autoimmune disease, I am a work in progress. My current issue is that I got mold in my body from working in my off-site jewelry office in the last year. The mold was growing in the wall behind where I sat. The mold is being stubborn, and it does not want to detox out of my body. This is a setback I didn't expect but am working to overcome. The mold has reminded me of the days when I first got ill with autoimmune disease and how it felt to feel lousy. This complication starts with healing my liver, which I am concentrating on now.

My first book is a wonderful guide for anyone struggling with chronic illness. We can do so much ourselves to encourage our bodies to heal that I had no idea about before getting sick. Finding the hundreds of toxins that I eliminated took five years of research, and the book gives others a jump-start to follow my lead to return to health themselves.

I just revised **It Feels Good to Feel Good, Learn to Eliminate Toxins, Reduce Inflammation and Feel Great Again** (2020) to include all chronic illnesses because I now know that this information is critical whether you have an autoimmune disease, cancer or heart disease. The book discusses all the things that you can do to change your lifestyle and feel great again. I learned that the body wants to heal; we need to give it the right building blocks so that it can do that.

In the revised book, I added new findings, and I included a chapter on Blue Zones because my information truly is for everyone, whether they are struggling with any chronic illness or not. Blue Zones are the National Geographic study about the five areas in the world where people live the longest and what people in these zones have in common. There is so much to learn from that study.

There are also new statistics that make toxins mind-boggling, and that proves my point. Keep in mind; it can take up to 20 years for inflammation to grow in the body to the tipping point of toxic load.

These are the statistics:

- 53% of our children are suffering from a chronic illness. This is a frightening statistic. Real food can make our children well, but the standard American diet is making them sick as hell.
- 30% are overweight.
- 16% of our children have learning disabilities.
- 11% of our children have asthma.
- 10% of our children have ADHD.
- 8% of our children have food allergies. There are no statistics on how many of our children have food sensitivities.
- 5% of our children have seizures.
- 2% of our male children have autism.
- By the time our children are five, they can have as many as 7 pounds of chemicals in their little bodies, according to Mark Hymen, MD, a leading

functional practitioner. No wonder they are getting ill, their little bodies cannot handle all these toxins.

- The new statistics state that a Millennial's health peaks at age 27 and then goes downhill.
- Gen-X'ers make it until age 37 before their health starts to decline. Still totally frightening.
- 10% of the population currently has diabetes.
- 33% of our population is pre-diabetic and will have diabetes in five years.
- 39% of our population has or will get cancer.
- 53 million Americans have an autoimmune disease, and they are mostly female. (This includes 1 in 5 females and 1 in seven males.)
- We are 37th in the world in health. And yet, we spend more on healthcare than any other country in the world. And our healthcare system is broken. Our healthcare system cannot keep up with the expense of the rapid rise of chronic illness in our country.
- Newborns are often being born with more than 287 toxins in their bodies, which they are inheriting from their mothers' bodies through the umbilical cord. Of the 287 chemicals that were detected in umbilical cord blood, we know that 180 cause cancer in humans or animals, 217 are toxic to the brain and nervous system, and 208 cause birth defects or abnormal development in animal tests.[2]
- Childhood asthma rose 300% in 40 years (GMO's exacerbate allergies)
- Childhood leukemia and brain cancer rose 40% in 40 years
- American couples dealing with fertility issues rose 20% in 10 years
- And Boomers, my generation, accept that they should live a life of pain and pills. And they are stuck; they don't want to change or be "deprived" by giving up what is making them sick.

What gives me hope from all of this?

- 52% OF ORGANIC BUYERS ARE MILLENIALS.
- It doesn't have to be this way. There are things each of us can do as individuals to change the tide.

Finally, our government is not protecting us. They are heavily influenced by Big Agriculture, Big Chemical, Big Pharmaceutical, and Big Food. I got angry about this in the beginning, but then I figured out that we need to join together and create the change we want to see. We have more power than we realize. The Institute of Responsible Technology says that a 5% shift in spending habits will begin to change what is happening. In the last three years, I have seen the needle slowly start to move.

My first book does not go far enough. It is discussing what I did in my immediate environment to clean up my life, my body, and my health.

Feeling Good: Living Low Toxin in Community and Everyday Life addresses the fact that we do not live in an isolated bubble, we live in a community, and living a low toxin life out in the community is more complicated. I have now been doing this, really, as self-defense, for more than three years. Living "clean" is something that I have figured out because I do not want the pain back, and I am a very social person. Community often means "eating." I interact fully now within my community in a way that does not interfere with my commitment to keep toxins as low in my life as possible, and in this book, I want to share all those tips. It is also common, once one gets one autoimmune disease, to get multiple autoimmune diseases, and I wanted to ensure that this didn't happen to me. In other words, I was very motivated to figure this out.

I now want to share this all with you. Once you clean up the toxins in your immediate life, these tips will help you avoid getting flares, they will help you minimize the pain, and they will help you minimize the progression of the diseases.

Living out in the community is swimming upstream. America eats the SAD, the Standard American Diet, which is loaded with toxins, synthetic ingredients, and fake food. The SAD does not offer our bodies any nutrients and instead serves up a healthy amount of synthetic ingredients that the body does not recognize as food. (SAD is processed food, fast food, factory meats, and junk food.)

Ever think about how a restaurant can have such a vast offering? Restaurants now often serve meals that they get in baggies, pre-prepared, that they microwave, and these meals are jampacked with nonfoods and synthetic ingredients without much food value. These prepared restaurant foods are loaded with toxins at every level, from the vegetables to the meats in their meals. And there are ingredients that have been added to all these foods that are unhealthy, and worst of all, addictive.

Even healthy restaurants often use unhealthy ingredients like their choice of oils. It's important to know what questions to ask and what to do to avoid these unhealthy ingredients.

Most restaurants use conventional produce, which means, if the produce is on the Dirty Dozen list, they are laden with nasty pesticide and herbicides that our bodies are not meant to process, and that are making us sick.

I had to figure this out; these foods made me ill. Yet, I refused to give up eating with my friends, family, and business associates.

I want to share all the tips I have discovered so that I can still thrive in my community, and I want you to be able to thrive too. It can be done; it just takes planning and some honest conversation. After a time, it becomes a way of life. So much of our social interaction takes place over food. Figuring out how to still participate in the social occasions of my life has been a growing experience.

I cook 90% of what we eat. I have learned a great deal over the last three years that I want to share. Food quality matters and I want to explain what that means and how I utilize that information. By cooking (or my hubby cooking), I can control what goes into my mouth and into my body. I want to share some of my tips about cooking most of our meals.

As a society, we have just gotten into bad habits. We are not making our health a priority. We are making convenience a priority. We need to go back to the way our great grandparents prepared their food.

It does not take that long to cook real organic live food, and the rewards are enormous.

There is a new definitive book out on toxins by Dr. Joseph Pizzorno, "The Toxin Solution: How Hidden Poisons in the Air, Water, Food, and Products We Use

Are Destroying Our Health--AND WHAT WE CAN DO TO FIX IT," HarperOne; Reprint edition (February 27, 2018), which gives all the scientific evidence that verifies what I discuss in my first book about toxins. In general, this book offers information so that when you adopt a low toxin life, you understand clearly why that is important for your health and the health of your family.

There is also important new information available about Epigenetics. They have discovered that no matter what genes you have inherited from your ancestors, you have some choice whether to turn on the switch and get that ailment or leave that switch off. It all has to do with lifestyle habits. Healthy habits keep the light switch for genetic diseases turned off. Living a life eating synthetic and toxic ingredients and surrounded by toxins turns the light switch on. If you have gotten the disease in your genetic makeup, you have a choice. I can't tell you how often someone has said to me, "I won't win. I inherited bad genetics. I was dealt a bad hand. I am going to get the disease that I inherited, so none of this matters." Au contraire. You control your environment, and your environment can control whether or not you get the disease.

Cleaning up the toxins in your life may not influence your health so much that you avoid getting whatever the disease IS in your genetics. There are other factors that influence your health. What it does do, is support your body so that it can build defenses against the disease and support your body to get through it. That in itself is worth all the tea in China.

One of the big push backs I get when I am out speaking about health is that eating healthy is expensive. I will share all my tips on buying healthy food on a budget. But think about it. Since it is now proven that toxins are creating ill health and disease, you can pay now, or you can pay later. As one organic farmer said, "Have you priced out the cost of cancer lately?" If you can avoid getting a chronic illness later in your life, it becomes very cost-efficient to eat as low toxin as possible and to eliminate the toxins in the rest of your life now.

I don't know where health insurance is going in this country but learning how to live low toxin is an insurance policy unto itself for your future and the future of your families. Our politicians are not discussing this because there is too much money flowing between Big Food, Big Ag, Big Pharma, and them. So, own this yourself, don't wait for someone else to protect you. You protect yourself and your family.

Finally, some people tell me that discussing toxins is boring. I had to laugh because when Dr. Joseph Pizzorno speaks at Integrative Medical Conferences, he hears the same thing. And he hears that it is depressing. All I can say is knowledge is power. And we need to know where the toxins are lurking so that we can "futureproof" our health. It isn't boring to stay healthy. And besides, "It Feels SO Good to Feel Good!"

Toxins may be an inconvenient truth, to borrow a phrase, but in the end, it can save your health and your mind. This allows you to grow old with grace and to prosper. Do you want to grow old with dementia and illness and pain, or do you want to thrive until the end? Since, at one point, I lost my health, I can tell you how I want to grow old, and everything you will learn about living low toxin is worth it in spades.

I am in a group on Facebook for a compounded drug called Naltrexone or LDN, and it is the closest thing to a "magic pill" that I have come across. It works extremely well for me, but I added it after I did everything in my power to clean up the toxins in my life and to lead a healthier life to eliminate my pain. This pill took me over the finish line to a pain-free life. If you struggle with chronic pain, I recommend that you investigate this medication with your doctor.

The drug is compounded (it comes from a compounding pharmacy), and although it works very well for me, it does not work as well for others in this Facebook group. You must be willing to clean up your environment and lifestyle if you want to live a pain-free life. Then this pill takes you over the finish line.

I know that we are all different, but I got to thinking, many in this group have not cleaned up their lives or adopted healthy habits. The medication implicitly states no alcohol on the label of the medication, and yet many are still drinking.

Health must start with healthy habits. And many in the group are getting more autoimmune conditions. This is not unusual if they still have a "leaky gut." Multiple syndrome autoimmune conditions are not unusual. The "magic" pill won't avoid that. The "magic" pill cannot be the only remedy. It's not that magic.

Eating organic live food of all the colors of the rainbow from a farm as close to you as possible and, if possible, in season, is the real magic pill. You control that. You don't need a prescription to buy that and eat that way. And if you remain healthy, your wellness bills, in the long run, will be much more affordable.

The Naltrexone does not take the place of healthy habits; it should be an addition to healthy habits. Perhaps this is the reason the pill works so well for me and not so well for others.

If you follow these tips and live a low toxin life, your body will celebrate. Learn to listen to your body, and it will make implementing these tips so worthwhile. And living a healthy life solves a multitude of health issues and gives your body a strong foundation to thrive.

One final thought and this is important. YOU are responsible for your health and for your child's health. Not your doctor, not your grocery store, not your farmers market, not your friends, not your druggist and certainly not your politician. You. And you are responsible for teaching your child good health so that they can grow up healthy and then teach their children all aspects of good health. Talk to your child about the importance of being a healthy influencer with their friends. The child's school is not responsible for their health, and again neither is their doctor. Many of these people play a role in health but own it yourself and be actively involved. It's your body and it's your child. Teach your child to take care of their body so that they have a happy place to live.

Put healthy habits into place now and reap the benefits. Nothing can beat healthy habits and a low toxin life.

To your health, with hugs, Cheryl

Introduction

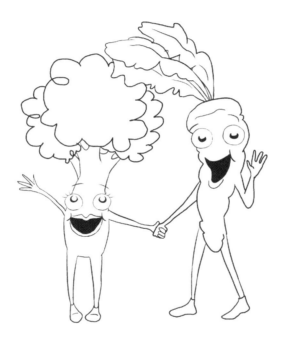

*"Anything is doable if you are willing to pay
the price and do the work to achieve it."*

DEBORAH STONE BATEMAN

If you are someone with chronic illness, you don't want the pain. If you hurt, you want to learn the tricks to keep that pain as low as possible. You don't want your chronic illness to progress. Your conventional MD's approach likely has you on multiple medications so that you can function as well as possible. Conventional MD's hear the complaint and match the pill. Some of your medications have downsides. You would love to find a better way.[3]

The first stage of this journey for me was identifying the toxins and what to replace them with that was lower toxin. I significantly lowered my toxic load.

My first book is very useful to lower your toxic load in your immediate environment—in your home and your immediate life. But we don't live isolated lives. We live in a community, and just because I stopped eating the SAD (Standard American Diet) didn't mean that I didn't want to spend time with my friends and my family. It didn't mean that I no longer wanted to go to my Chamber of Commerce meetings, which meet over food. It didn't mean that I no longer wanted to entertain or to go to parties or dinner at loved one's homes. I am only married for five years. My hubby and I love to travel, which also presented food complications. This book is about how I figured out how I can still live in a community and enjoy all the people that I love and how I do all the things that I want to do without raising my toxic parameters.

This book is about stage two. This book is about everything that I have learned since I wrote book one, **It Feels Good to Feel Good, Learn to Eliminate Toxins, Reduce Inflammation, and Feel Great Again**.[4]

The good news is that it's never too late to start making health-conscious choices. Once you begin good habits, you start to feel terrific, and you want to keep feeling that way. I have more energy; I am not fatigued when I wake up in the morning; I have discovered boundless energy. I have learned how to control my stress, and I have better coping mechanisms. Once you start to make better health choices, you extend that to all areas of your life.

Amazingly, we can eat poorly for years and "abuse" our bodies, and yet, our bodies can still heal! I chose that I never wanted to live a life of pain again, so I started to explore how to maintain healthy habits in all areas of my life.

I believe that health begins with "clean" food and a healthy gut, so maintaining that has become the objective of how John and I now live. We love to go to farmer's markets. We love to talk to the farmers. There are different "healthy" things available at different markets, and shopping these markets became fun things for us to explore.

My husband, John, got more involved with a Dao philosophy organization and started exercising with the Mago group and doing meditation. I practice daily gratitude before I start my day. I started to explore different daily exercises I could do that would keep my stress level under control and keep me healthy. And some of the exercises I share are things John and I have learned through the Dao Group we practice with.

I am still an "A" personality, but I release the steam regularly during the day, like an instant pot, before it becomes too high to blow. As a result, my cortisol levels have balanced out. My chronic fatigue is pretty much gone. John and I do read different books, but we are on parallel paths, and we discuss what we have learned at the end of each day. We continue to grow in the same direction from different approaches.

Food is a big deal. Eliminating all the non-food from our diet is a big deal. Changing what we eat has changed our bodies and how good we feel. Now that we know the difference good quality food makes to our bodies, we want to maintain that even when we are out with friends or family. Food Quality Matters. I am particularly careful because I don't want to trigger my disease, but John and I are equally committed to eating quality food no matter where we are and who has joined us. These have been learned skills that I now want to share with you. We love socializing; it just doesn't change what kind of food we want to put into our bodies. We have had a total mindset change, which makes this a no brainer now.

It's easy to control what goes into my mouth and my body if I am cooking. It is not so easy to swim upstream and eat differently than the rest of America when I get out of my house.

And some people believe that how John and I eat is "boring" and that eliminating toxins and living differently from others is bazaar. I have tried to make toxins as fun as possible, and you will see it in the art at the beginning of each chapter. I have 36 characters now that I have developed to encourage others and especially children, to eat differently and to embrace their veggies and healthy habits.

In this book, I talk about how quickly different cells in our body are replaced. John and I have made a decision to replace them with healthy cells because they are built from healthy building blocks.

I know what it feels like to feel lousy, and I don't ever want to go back to that. The SAD (Standard American Diet) is using the wrong grade gasoline in my body. It was chugging along but headed towards disaster. All the lights came on in the dashboard of my body. Had I not reacted when I did, my disease would have progressed past the point of no return.

Before I got sick, I don't think that I found food and how to eat confusing. I didn't think about it. Grabbing something fast was so easy, whether it was a frozen meal with synthetic chemicals, a box of cookies with GMO flour and tons of sugar or fructose, or a hamburger from Mc Donald's made with non-food.

When I was told by a nutritionist to start eating real live fruits and veggies, bells went off in my head. It made sense, and from that day forward, I no longer wanted that "other" stuff. I always enjoyed eating veggies and fruits; they just weren't my first choice. And eliminating my sensitivities and eating real quality food made a difference in how good I felt in a very short period. It was worth it! I always want to feel this way now.

I had to break my addiction to sugar. The sugar calls your name. You keep going back for more, no matter how full you are. Before you can truly enjoy the taste and the power of live food, you must break the hold of the sugar on your body. And synthetic ingredients and MSG in processed foods are also addictive and have the same effect on the body. Then you must eliminate GMOs. I have a full explanation in my first book, but BT toxin and Glyphosate are toxins harming your body. Once you get away from all these toxic ingredients, it's a whole new game. All those things, sugar, GMOs, synthetic ingredients, MSG, fast food, processed food, take away choice because they are addictive. Breaking the hold these non-food ingredients have on our body is food freedom and the path to health.

Once you do that, you begin to eat to nourish your body. You begin to thrive on the taste of a good tomato, that was organically grown, or an organic berry that came directly from the farm. You don't eat from compulsion, but for vitality, the vitality of the plant that gives your body the life energy to function. It becomes a different mindset, and your physical body starts to thrive. You can "feel" the difference. Your body starts to celebrate.

I never doubted that I could return to wellness. I did a ton of research when my Mother first got Multiple System Atrophy, and she was only supposed to survive her disease two years, but she lived another 10. I knew if I set my mind to it, I would also find the information that I needed to return to wellness myself. I didn't do it all alone, I found a fantastic functional MD who got me where I wanted to go, and helped me heal, but I started at home with the basics and then she took me the rest of the way over the finish line. And I never doubted that I would figure out how to eat my new, clean and healthy diet out in a community, but this has taken quite a bit of trial and error. If these tips can make your life easier, then I want to share them with you.

John, my hubby, was on board with being on a wellness journey with me from the beginning. I met him eight years ago because the guy that I was in a relationship with didn't like it that I was sick, and we broke up. Since I was in my 60's, I went online to an old fogie dating site and put out feelers for someone who wanted to go on a "Get Well Journey" with me. I had lots of other requirements as well, like intelligence and ethics, and John answered in 3 days, and he only lived 10 minutes away from me. Funny how the universe works. He had just lost his wife of 42 years to cancer, and he had gained a ton of weight. He said he wanted to go on a get-well journey with me right from the beginning, and that it would be wonderful to do it together. And, he was a statistician, with a minor in English literature. My major was English literature. He did shopping-cart analysis, and other forms of data analysis, I was a former department store retailer and had my own jewelry business. We were opposite sides of the coin to embark on this new adventure headed in the same direction. And I lucked out. What a lovely supportive man I married. He wants me to be happy, and he lovingly supports me in every way. If I am busy writing or doing something to promote my business now, he will plan and do the cooking. He edits my videos. He reads my chapters as the grammar and spelling police. He even will read a book on a subject I am studying and send me the most important phrases from the book for me to consider using in my writing.

As a result of our *Get-Well Journey*, both of our lives are significantly better. We have not given anything up that matters to us. We still get together with loved ones to feast, but what we feast on is different. We still enjoy the meal, but it has the added advantage of being a gift to our company or the people that we love that we are sharing it with. The way we eat now is a new way to relish the good company of our loved ones and a new way to continue feeling fantastic. We never preach or judge, but we are committed to staying true to our way of eating. It oozes out of us. It does "Feel Good," and we intend to maintain that. And if you want to eat differently around us, that's ok too. It just isn't going to change our commitment to our health and what we put into our mouth.

This book is about our total change in lifestyle. We are not on a temporary diet; I understand now that this is for life. And John and I live well and are not hindered in any way from living the life that we want to live. We have just had to figure it all out. Our goal now is to live to old age, feeling great, and keeping our minds healthy. It's so worth it to feel good. We are happy; we are well. Life is good.

I have included a chapter on how the toxins and poisons are impacting our fur babies. When I met John, I had three beloved kitties. I have always had pets, and the joke with my friends was, in their next life, they wanted to come back as one of my pets. Before these guys, my two previous cats lived to 20 and 24.

But I lost these sweethearts at 12, 14 and 16. While I was busy working on my health, I was not paying attention to the fact that, although I was feeding my kitties the same food that I had always fed my pets, the food had dramatically changed. It, too, was loaded with GMOs and BT Toxin. It also was loaded with Glyphosate (Roundup). The 12-year-old died of mouth cancer, and the 14 and 16-year-old kitties died of kidney disease and probably cancer.

Had I had dogs, I probably would have missed that just taking them on a walk would have been exposing them to herbicides and pesticides along the path.

I want to make you aware of what is going on. I miss my three babies a lot, and I feel bad that I didn't figure it out before I lost them so early. You will find an entire section on our pets and their health in this book (Part IX).

What is happening to our pet companions is exactly the same thing that is happening to us. Food quality matters for them too. They need to eat species-specific food with the right building blocks for their bodies. They also struggle with leaky gut. Owners are looking for the magic pill to keep them healthy as well. The magic pill is their food and is in not allowing them to be over medicated and over-vaccinated. The magic pill is in keeping their environment "low toxin."

How we are looking at health is changing. Just because you get certain DNA and genetics is a blueprint that you inherit, doesn't mean that you are going to get that same disease that has always been in your family. Your lifestyle and what you eat, in other words, your environment, makes a difference as to whether you turn that light switch on, or you leave it off. The toxins go into the cell, corrupt it, and turn your genetics on, not the other way around. You control so much. If I can convince you that you are not a victim and that you need to own your own body and your health, then you have a better chance to live long and thrive.

My tips are for anyone who wants a healthier lifestyle, a get-well journey of their own. I included the highlights of my chapter on the Blue Zones from the revised version on my first book because we all need to go on a get-well journey, or it will become a journey to disease in short order. Take a moment and go back and look at the statistics in my Preface. They are frightening.

The Blue Zones are the areas in the world where people live the longest without disease and dementia. Your toxic load can take as long as 20 years to creep up before it topples over the top. America is on a collision course with disease. Our health care system is broken because our food system is broken. Our lifestyle is broken. Our environment is broken. The products we regularly use have poisons in them. We are poisoning the earth, which is then poisoning us. Everyone needs to pay attention to eating real quality food and eliminating all the poisons that are in other areas of our life. The Blue Zone study has proven that this is possible, and it connects the dots as to why this is important.

If you don't need what I am suggesting now, and you don't pay attention to it, you will most likely need it somewhere down the road. And unfortunately, that will probably be sooner than later. I want to encourage you to change NOW so that you don't end up like I did, sick as the dickens.

Most importantly, I have written several chapters on our children's' health and things we can do to improve it. Their little bodies cannot process all of the toxins that they are encountering on a daily basis. Today the statistic is that 53% of our children have a chronic disease. If we don't make a commitment to clean up how we are living now, what will the statistic be ten years or twenty-five years from now? We can't wait. Change must happen now.

I am proud to be 71. I feel good. Life is good. I am responsible for me. I know I am going to die, but I choose to live as healthy as I can for as long as I can. And if my tips help you do the same, then my getting sick was worth it, for both of us. To our health!

"When diet is wrong, medicine is of no use; when diet is correct, medicine is of no need."

ANCIENT AYURVEDIC PROVERB

Part I

Something You Need to Know

Chapter 1

What We Have Learned from Blue Zones

Why They Should Motivate You to a Cleaner Toxin-free Life

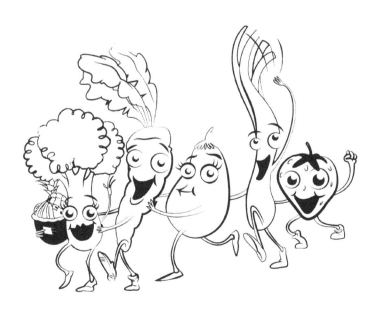

THE BIG TAKEAWAYS ON BLUE ZONES:[5]

- *The Blue Zone study by National Geographic is important to all of us as a "blueprint" for our future health.*

- *Blue Zones are the five areas in the world with the highest human longevity, where it is common to live over 100 and to remain healthy and vibrant until the end.*

- *Nine key elements contribute to human longevity: Community, Diet, Cooking, Drinking, Treats, Mind, Sleep, Movement, and Life Purpose.*

I wrote about Blue Zones in the revision of my first book, **It Feels Good to Feel Good, Learn to Eliminate Toxins, Reduce Inflammation and Feel Great Again**. I feel so strongly about this information; I decided to also include the information in this book.

If you, your children and the other people in your life are healthy, then why should you care about toxins and the quality of your food?

I wrote this chapter because I often hear this objection when I am speaking to groups. It is part of the "toxins are boring" conversation and part of the "I don't intend to change because nothing is wrong with my health" conversation. It is also part of the "I like the convenience of fast food and processed food, and I don't intend to cook" conversation." And it's partially because people don't understand that toxic Load is something that builds up over time. It could take 20 years to build up and topple over the top. *You might not be as healthy as you think*.

These people don't open their ears to even listen to what I have to say. Discussing this research is my shot to reposition the information so that, perhaps, they can "hear" me.

We can all learn a great deal from observing Blue Zones.

Blue Zones[6] are the five areas in the world with the highest human longevity, where it is common to live over 100 and to remain healthy and vibrant until the end. Quality of life in these zones is very high. It is a project sponsored by National Geographic.

There are now nine more communities across America that are electing to be Blue Zones. Fort Worth, Texas; Manhattan Beach, California and surrounding beach cities; Klamath, Oregon; Albert Lea, Minnesota; Southwest Florida; Iowa; Dodge County, Wisconsin; and Pottawatomie County, Oklahoma have all now elected to be Blue Zones communities.

What would motivate you to pay attention to the results in Blue Zones? Why would this matter to you? And by discovering this information, will you change?

Toxic Load can take 20 years to build up in your body. Toxic Load becomes Inflammation. Inflammation becomes Chronic Disease. The chronic disease could be autoimmune disease, or cancer or heart disease. Chronic illness begins with toxins and Inflammation. So long term, this information can save your health.

Convenience is trumping health, and our nation's health is showing the result. No wonder the United States ranks 37th in the world in health, our healthcare system is broken, and 53% of our children have chronic illnesses.

You want to eat the Standard American Diet. You want to eat what everyone else eats. Food is at the center of social relationships, so you don't want to eat differently than everyone else. You want to eat for convenience, and you don't want to go to the trouble to eat differently. You certainly don't want to cook.

You don't care about the chemicals being sprayed on our food or the poisons that we are eating on and in our food.

But let me ask you, what good is it for you to grow old if you are uncomfortable in your body, if your body has cancer or heart disease, or if you are one of the millions of people with autoimmune disorders? What good is it, if you are struggling with a lot of pain every morning, or if, in old age, you have lost your mind to dementia?

Don't you want to grow old and feel great, and still able to enjoy living your life? Don't you want your children to grow old and to be healthy? For the first time, your children may not live as long as you, and their last years are not projected to be pretty.

This information is important.

Don't you want to have quality of life as you age?

Here's what National Geographic has discovered from the Blue Zones.

Some key elements contribute to long term health and healthy longevity in a Blue Zone Community:

1   Community

    All Blue Zones have strong communities. Some are people that have been connected for life; most have a faith-based connection. Sometimes multi-generations live together. These communities share a sense of purpose with their members. They are people that support each other throughout life. Finding a supportive community that shares your healthy values is important.

2   Diet

    All the Blue Zones eat a healthy, low-toxin diet. Most are vegetarian, with some wild fish, and sometimes very small portions of pastured meat twice a week. Common foods that are eaten in Blue Zones are organic and include olive oil, lots of greens, coffee, chickpeas, legumes, green tea, tomatoes, turmeric, sweet potatoes, salmon, squash and avocados.

3   Cook

    Eating out is celebratory only. Food is made in the home and eaten in their family community. Food is never eaten standing up or in the car. Plates are made in the kitchen and taken to the table. People in blue zones stop eating when they are 80% full.

4   Drink

The people in Blue Zones drink water. They don't drink sodas with sugar or fake sugar. And at the end of the day, they have one glass of wine.

5   Treats

Blue Zones keep healthy food accessible and ready to eat on upper shelves in their fridge at eye level. Junk food is eliminated. You eat what you see, and you eat what is convenient. Make freshly cut veggies and fruit the foods that are easy to eat.

6   Mind

Blue Zones have people with active minds. They are constantly learning, be it a new language, a new musical instrument or new science. Often people in blue zones meditate.

7   Sleep

People in Blue Zones get seven or more hours of sleep. The bedroom is only used for sleep or sex. No TV, No phone. No clock. The room is kept cool.

8   Movement

People in Blue Zones move naturally. They walk everywhere. They ride bikes for transportation. They get up and down to change the TV channel; they do outdoor chores, and they garden. They have pets that they walk.

9   They all have a life purpose.

People in Blue Zones have a passion and a mission for what they want to accomplish in the world.

To sum it all up, people living in Blue Zones have healthy social communities; they have strong family bonds; they have no time urgency; they eat a plant-based diet; they do not smoke; they eat legumes; they have low alcohol intake; they eat nuts. They garden. They have turmeric in their diet. They eat nutrient-rich diets. They all pre-plated their food in the kitchen so that they don't overeat. They eat off smaller plates.

They have significantly less cancer, heart disease, autoimmune disease, and almost no dementia. Blue Zone communities are places where it is common for people to live to 100; they suffer a fraction of the diseases that kill people in the rest of the world, and they enjoy many more years of good health.

Their smallest meal is their evening meal. They all enjoy some natural physical activity. They live low-stress lives. They all enjoy some form of faith.

They eat chemical-free. They live in clean environments. They support each other.

Does this information resonate with you? Don't wait until you are sick and tired of being sick and tired. Clean up your life now. You only have one body. Honor it and take care of it, and it will serve you well. And by the by, don't give me that bull that you have bad genes. In most instances you have the power to turn that switch on or to leave it off. Having something in your genetics does not mean that you are going to get it. The reverse of that is if you have good genes, they will not protect you from future disease in your life if you don't live clean lifestyles. You make all the difference with your body. You hold the power. Own it and feel great for the rest of your life.

Blue Zone findings are the same things I discuss in my book; ***It Feels Good to Feel Good, Learn to Eliminate Toxins, Reduce Inflammation, and Feel Great Again***. *These are pointers for people with chronic illness to adopt. They are just as important for YOU, whether you are sick or well.*

Part II

Food Quality Matters

Chapter 2

What's your deal with Food?

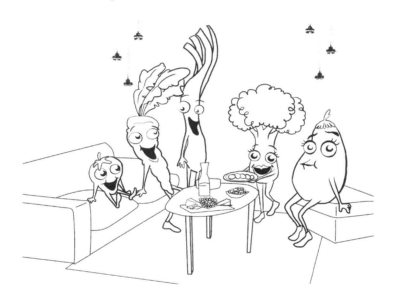

As we move forward to the importance of food quality, I think it is important to contemplate what Food means to you.

What is Food to you?[7]

- Is Food love?
- Is Food community?
- Is Food energy?
- Is Food pleasure?
- Is Food sustenance?
- Is Food power?
- Is Food happiness?
- Is Food life?
- Is Food nutrients?
- Is Food compassion?
- Or is Food junk, chemicals, toxins, pesticides, herbicides, and "fast and easy"?

I ask, because if I told you, "if you changed how you ate and it could cure your pain," would you do it?

If you ate to live rather than lived to eat, what would that look like?

If you ate nutrient-dense foods and food for sustenance, can it still bring you pleasure? You know that it could bring you health.

Does that resonate with you?

Your body needs nutrients for life. Feeding your body chemicals cannot sustain you, which is why we see so much disease.

- 10% of the population currently has diabetes.
- 33% of our population is pre-diabetics and will have diabetes in 5 years.
- 39% of our population has or will get cancer
- Fifty-three million Americans have an autoimmune disease, mostly females. (This includes one in five females and one in seven males)
- If you eat more nutrient-dense foods and could avoid all of this, would you do it?

Does this resonate?

*"Why do you do what you do when
you know what you know?"*

DR. LIBBY WEAVER

Can you eat nutrient-dense foods that still bring you pleasure?

What would that look like?

Could you show love in ways other than food?

If you are eating differently from others in your community, does it mean that you can't join them?

Could you enjoy your community from other perspectives?

What if clean food could still bring you pleasure?

If you reframed food to use real ingredients with real nutrients and still had yummy things to eat, would that bring you pleasure?

Could that bring you the same happiness?

If Food made you healthy, could it bring you more happiness?

I am here to tell you, yes, it can. Don't wait until you get sick to discover "real food." Eliminate all the ingredients that you can't pronounce. Eliminate the foods with chemical names that you don't know what they are. If you don't know what they are, neither does your body. This includes ingredients like "natural flavors." Do you know what that is? I don't and believe it or not, sometimes it is MSG.

Buy live food, organic when necessary. Cook. Sit around the table at home with your loved ones, Eat plants. Choose from all the colors of the rainbow. They each have some wonderful gift to give to you. Eat seasonally as much as possible.

You must discover what food means to you, and then you need to reframe food so that you fill the same emotions with healthy substitutions. Food can make you well. Food can keep you well, or food can make you sick as hell.

Avoid all the chemicals; avoid all the fake ingredients, and most of your health battles are over. Your body will begin to heal itself. Real chemical-free food heals.

Good health doesn't have to be difficult. It isn't about deprivation. Good health is about the joy of finding the life that you have always wanted but didn't know how to get.

Good health is about reframing what you have been eating and making different choices that have the benefit of feeding your body lovely nutrients. Real food has the added benefit of bringing you vitality. It will make you glow. These foods will highlight your beauty.

I read a product marketing slogan not too long ago that made an impression on me. "I eat nutritious, delicious, and nothing suspicious."[8] This phrase sums it all up for me, and it should also sum it up for you.

No more Standard American Diet for me. And I am worth it.

You are only one decision away
from a different life.

UNKNOWN

Chapter 3

Health Begins in the Kitchen

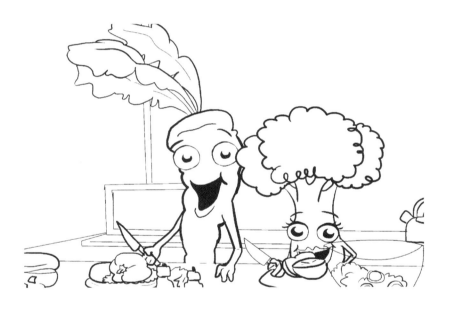

Each color of veggie and fruit offer different gifts to the body, but the real miracle is that all the phytonutrients and photo nutrients work together to create health in your body

THE BIG TAKEAWAYS ON HEALTH BEGINS IN THE KITCHEN:[9]

- *The body wants to heal. We just need to give it the right building blocks for it to be able to do that.*

- *Color is crucial to health. All the colors work together in synergy to heal us.*

- *Eat organic fruits and vegetables from a farm as close to you as possible and eat in-season for maximum nutrition.*

- *I have learned it doesn't matter whether you choose to eat Paleo, Vegetarian, or Vegan. The important part is that three-quarters of what you eat are vegetables and fruits. If they are on the Dirty Dozen, then make sure you eat them organic.*

- *The Magic pill we have all been looking for is in the colors of our fruits and vegetables. It will never be a pharmaceutical.*

- *Find as many ways as possible to incorporate multiple colors of fruits and veggies in your daily food plan. Feel their goodness flow through your veins.*

- *Your body will celebrate.*

The importance of eating color

Since I got sick and started eating real live food, 90% of which I am cooking myself, I have learned three valuable lessons:

1. The body wants to heal. We need to give it the right building blocks to be able to do that. Just like computers, garbage in, garbage out. Eating nutrient-rich foods gives our bodies the building blocks it needs to rebuild.

2. Color is crucial to health. All the colors work together in synergy to heal us. If we were to take the same nutrients isolated in capsules, they would not only not work the same way, but new studies have shown that the nutrients in isolation might create harm to the body. Eaten together, in their natural state, they create health. Nature and the greater plan never cease to amaze me.

3   It is so important to eat food that comes from a local farm. Every week, you must "eat all of the colors of the rainbow." You must cook your own food, as frequently as possible, so that you control the ingredients that go into your body. This way, you get maximum nutrition, and it all works together for the greater good of your body.

Now, I recognize how lucky I am. I live in both California and Arizona, and I have a greater abundance of fresh produce direct from the farm to purchase. I have suggestions that I will present later in this book as to what to do if you are not as lucky as I am and live in areas where fresh veggies are not as abundant. Just keep in mind how important these concepts are right now, and then we will figure out how everyone can participate. Right now, I want to discuss color and what each color has to offer to us when eaten in synergy.

And I have learned it doesn't matter whether you choose to eat Paleo, Vegetarian or Vegan, the important part is that three-quarters of what you eat are vegetables and fruits. You do not need vast amounts of animal meat if you choose to eat it. I keep it to the size of the palm of my hand. And I try to eat vegetables for breakfast, lunch, and dinner. Eating lots of fruits and vegetables makes my body sing, and now that I pay attention to what my body is saying to me, I know that this is the right way for me to eat.

In the last eighteen months, I have done more than 100 podcasts. One of my favorites was with Billionaire Brown. When I told him I often eat spinach for breakfast (often with a poached egg), he kept saying, "Spinach for breakfast? For breakfast? Spinach?" It got very funny because of the tone in his voice. Yep, spinach for breakfast. I love, love, love it. And why the heck not? Spinach is loaded with goodness and with iron. Yum. Add some diced organic tomato on top, and it's one yummy breakfast.

I eat for my body now. And I am rewarded for it.

I always hated to diet because I hated trying to follow all the rules. I am a person that likes to think outside the box and needs freedom of choice. Eating healthy is so much easier. You learn the basics and then use your

freedom to eat within those basics. And your body responds so positively. It is fantastic!

We need a rainbow of nutrients and colors.

The variety of vitamins, minerals, antioxidants, and phytochemicals in fruits and vegetables have enormous healing powers. Many of these gifts show up in their distinctive colors.

Eating a diversity of colorful foods can be an easy way to get the complete range of vitamins and minerals your body needs to thrive.

The advice to "eat the rainbow" is important for kids. Kids especially need a diversity of foods in their diets, but so do adults. (Kids use their parents as models, so you must eat healthy for them as well as for yourself.)

The gut microbiome is incredibly important to your overall health, and it is best to have a varied population. The best way to achieve this variety for the gut is to consume a diet filled with assorted foods. Studies have found that the types of food you consume have a strong influence on the environment in the gut. And never forget, if the fruit or vegetable is on the dirty dozen list, buy and eat it organic. Remember that this list is updated every year. Go to the back of this book to see what is currently on the only organic list. You can also always find it on my website https://cherylmhealthmuse.com/author-and-book-info/dirty-dozen-plus-clean-15/

You never need a healthy dose of herbicides and pesticides with your food. To learn more about how GMO's and conventionally sprayed produce impact our bodies, go back and read those chapters in **It Feels Good to Feel Good, Learn to Eliminate Toxins, Reduce Inflammation and Feel Great Again**.[10]

If you eat diverse foods, there is a lower risk of food allergy and intolerance. When you eat the same food, again and again, you increase your risk of developing a food intolerance or allergy to that food.

I have 15 food sensitivities that I must eat around, and this certainly was the case with chicken and me. I ate so much chicken; I used to joke that I was going to cluck at any moment. Well, now it has become a sensitivity, and it creates serious inflammation in my body, I need to be careful not to eat so much beef that I begin to Moo. Ha! No, now I have learned to eat lesser amounts of my meat, and I do eat all the different types available, and only if they are pastured and eat their species-specific diet. I realize we are discussing fruits and vegetables here, but the same rules exist. Always have diversity in the foods you eat.

> Note—Researchers determined that a decrease in food diversity between 6 and 12 months of age has an association with food sensitivities and/ or allergies.

There are many companies out there now that are selling fruit and veggie powders that you drink. Ok, if you can't find that actual food, I can see the benefits of drinking this. However, what I want is for you to eat the veggie, fruit, and fiber all together for maximum nutrition. Eat the whole food. Yes, preferably, it should be organic, and it should be organic if it is on the dirty dozen list that's a must but eat the entire food. This way, the food is not processed. You are eating it as close to nature as possible. The Universe made that food perfect exactly the way it is. I would only drink the powders if the real food were not available.

Why is it important to eat all the colors of the rainbow?

- All the colors of real live foods have gifts for the body. Research shows that different colors are good for different conditions of the human body.
- There are variations of nutrients in each of the colors. This is something that most people don't know.
- The typical diet provides more than 25,000 bioactive food components.
- Phytochemicals, also referred to as phytonutrients, are found in fruits, vegetables, whole grains, legumes, beans, herbs, spices, nuts, and seeds and are classified according to their chemical structures and functional properties.

- Each color in fruits and vegetables is caused by specific phytonutrients, which are natural chemicals that help protect plants from germs, bugs, the sun's harmful rays, and other threats.
- Each color indicates an abundance of specific nutrients.[11]
- Eating all the colors of the rainbow creates a varied population of healthy gut bacteria.
- Specific foods, not just diet, have a huge influence on your microbiome.
- Eat as close to the farm as possible. Where your food is grown, impacts the "gifts" that each food has to offer.
- Variety is key because of the synergy of the different phytochemicals working together.
- Variety in eating all the colors lowers inflammation. This helps prevent many of our chronic diseases.
- Eating all the colors of the rainbow neutralizes free radicals and lowers oxidative stress.

Your diet must include a variety of multiple foods in each color group.

It's Important to Eat the Rainbow. Diversity is Key.

8 out of 10 people in the U.S. are falling short in virtually every color category of phytonutrients.[12]

Based on the report:

- 69% of Americans are falling short in green phytonutrients
- 78% of Americans are falling short in red phytonutrients
- 86% of Americans are falling short in white phytonutrients
- 88% of Americans are falling short in purple and blue phytonutrients
- 79% of Americans are falling short in yellow and orange phytonutrients

Eating all the colors of the rainbow creates a healthy gut.[13]

A rich and diverse diet of whole foods offers the best combination of micronutrients and phytochemicals. Eating these is the best way to get your vitamins and minerals and your phytochemicals. Without these nutrients, we face poor health, disease, obesity, and more.

You still might need to supplement to get all the minerals and vitamins you need. But FOOD QUALITY MATTERS and eating high-quality real food gives your body most of the building blocks necessary to keep it functioning at an optimal level.

When it comes to food, crowd out with color rather than eat with restrictive rules.

Color is sustainable, creative and engaging, whereas rules are restrictive, demanding, and exhaustive.

DEANNA MINICH, PH.D.——FACEBOOK 10/12/19

Note—I gave a class on Food Quality Matters early last year (2019), and one of the classes was on color. The information listed in this chapter started with my interest in Dr. Deanna Minich's work and reading her books. She is all about color, and her work inspired me to learn more and to incorporate her information into my healthy habits and talks. The information in this chapter is a compilation from reading a variety of sources as well from:

Deanne Minich, Ph.D.
Dr. Josh Axe
Dr. David Jocker
Disabled World
Food Revolution Ocean Robbins
Food Matters website
Food for Life
Ohio State—Your Plan for Health

I know that my body rejoices both mentally and physically when I incorporate all the colors of the rainbow into my diet. For more information, Start with reading Deanna Minich's work. **The Rainbow Diet: A Holistic Approach to Radiant Health Through Foods and Supplements** by Minich Ph.D. CNS, Deanna M. Conari Press; 1 edition; Jan 1, 2018

There are physical and emotional responses to color.

Serving food from all the color groups enhances your eating experience, encourages your children to eat a healthier variety, stimulates the brain, and creates both physical and emotional responses.

Colorful foods are very appealing to the senses, making food fun as well as nutritious, and it brings pleasure on a variety of different levels.

By adding a variety of color to your meals, your food also feeds all of your senses, as it feeds your body. I love color, and color feeds my soul. Even in my years designing jewelry, I was known for my color and never enjoyed working in "white" gems-diamonds or cubic zirconia, when I switched to silver. The white stones exist to enhance the beauty of color for me. Color makes me happy, so creating colorful meals works for me as well on a variety of levels.

If you have children, it will encourage them to eat healthier food. With color, you can create fun plates for your children, and the goal is to encourage them to eat real live food. Color plays an important part in that.

So, let's talk about the different colors, what fruits and vegetables come in those colors, and what the gifts of each color are to our bodies. I am going to discuss them in isolated groups, but remember, they must work together to create maximum health.

Red

Fruits and vegetables available in the red family.

Blood oranges
Cherries
Cranberries
Pink/red grapefruit
Pomegranate
Radicchio
Radishes
Raspberries
Red apples
Red beets
Red cabbage
Red grapes
Red onions
Red pears
Red peppers
Red potatoes
Rhubarb
Strawberries
Tomatoes
Watermelon

Red foods fortify your immune system.

When your immune system is working properly, it is your natural defense system. Red foods fight against the common cold and the Flu, then bolster and protect your body from chronic illness and cancer.

Compounds in strawberries, cherries, and red berry fruits are important for cardiovascular health and brain health.

Tomatoes have lycopene, important for cardiovascular health and cancer prevention.

There is a theory, currently being studied, that cholesterol is scurvy of the arteries. To prevent cholesterol from sticking to artery walls, you need vitamin C. C is also important to resist infection, and it supports immune function. Berries have lots of vitamins C and E.

These are some of the other gifts of red foods:

- Red foods protect your eyes from macular degeneration.
- Red foods protect you from strokes and cardiovascular disease. They lower blood pressure.
- Phytochemicals in some red foods help prevent cancer. Red foods soak up damaging free radicals.
- Red foods are great for improving memory function.
- They help create a healthy urinary tract. (For any woman that has struggled with urinary tract infections like I have, you know the wonder of cranberry juice to help reverse the infection. I start drinking cranberry at the first sign of trouble.)
- Red foods help people with arthritis reduce joint pain.
- Red foods help improve skin. Good skin and skin diseases are an inside job, cleaning up your gut, and eating all the colors of the rainbow will heal a multitude of issues from eczema, psoriasis, to acne. And it will slow aging to the skin. (See my chapter "Beauty is an Inside Job." Chapter 14)

Getting your phytonutrients from whole foods is best. Taking phytonutrients, like lycopene and beta-carotene, **in supplement form, may <u>increase</u> the risk of cancer**. But consuming these phytonutrients in whole-food form, like tomato sauce, has been found to decrease the risk of cancer.

Pretty interesting stuff.

Careful: apples, strawberries, red peppers, red potatoes, and tomatoes are on the dirty dozen list, so please buy organic. Strawberries are the dirtiest because they grow so close to the ground. (Billionaire Brown, on his podcast, kept saying

STRAWBERRIES? Please tell me Not Strawberries. Yep. They are the worst. That doesn't mean you don't get to eat strawberries; you just make sure that you eat them organic.)

There are also GMO apples and tomatoes on the market, trust me, you don't want those chemicals in your body either. The toxins negate any benefit you would get from the veggie and fruit, so please protect yourself and buy them organic. In Chapter 5, I discuss how to buy healthy food on a budget, so use those tips to buy the best possible produce for your health.

Now let's look at Orange foods.

Orange

Orange foods include:

Apricots
Cantaloupe
Carrots (help prevent cancer)
Kumquat
Mango
Nectarines
Orange bell pepper
Oranges the pith is loaded with fiber and nutrients
Papaya
Peaches
Persimmons
Pumpkin
Sweet potatoes (skin loaded with vitamin C)
Yams

Orange foods also fortify your immune system.

Orange foods have carotenoids, folate, potassium, and vitamin C.

- Orange plants provide a source of beta-carotene and other phytonutrients that have potent antioxidant activity.
- They protect sexual organs in both men and women.
- They help balance hormones.
- Orange foods are also high in vitamin C and Quercetin.
- Orange and yellow fruits and vegetables are rich in vitamin C and carotenoids, including beta-carotene. Some carotenoids, most notably beta-carotene, convert to vitamin A within the body, which helps promote healthy vision and cell growth.
- Citrus fruits contain a unique phytonutrient called hesperidin, which helps to increase blood flow. This has important health ramifications. *If you tend to get cold hands and feet, eating an orange a day may help keep your hands and feet warm*. More importantly, consuming citrus may also reduce your risk of stroke.
- The colorful and healthful plant pigments beta-carotene, beta-cryptoxanthin, and lycopene are more bioavailable from papaya than from raw tomato and carrot.[14]
- Orange foods fortify the immune system.
- They reduce age-related Macular-Degeneration.
- They reduce the risk of cancer and heart disease.
- They help lower LDL cholesterol.
- They prevent scurvy.
- The prevent rickets.
- They help eliminate constipation.
- They help promote brain development in infants.
- They provide a remedy for the common cold and cough.
- They are a rich source of vitamin C.
- They help lower blood pressure.
- They promote collagen formation and healthy joints.
- They fight harmful free radicals.
- They encourage alkaline balance.

- They improve brain function.
- They work with magnesium and calcium for healthy bones.
- They help relieve muscle cramps.
- Turmeric (Curcumin) lowers chronic pain and heals inflammation. I love this one, and it is what I now take for pain.
- They encourage collagen production, protecting joints.

As an aside—I heard a story from a farmer when I first started investigating organic vs. GMOs and conventional farming. He told me that carrots were not originally orange. When Bugs Bunny appeared in a color Warner Bros cartoon eating a carrot ("this way to Cucamonga"), his carrot was orange, and that started a huge demand for orange carrots. He told me the story to convince me that foods had been engineered for a very long time.

I share this story, but it's part of the hype of the chemical industry to convince you that GMO's have been around forever. The story is completely skewed.

That is true, carrots have been engineered, but only to something that would have occurred naturally in nature. They weren't genetically modified to be some Frankenfood that either has B.T. Toxin in it or has been doused with Roundup, which is Glyphosate, which has recently lost three lawsuits because it causes cancer. GMO foods are not engineered; they are modified to be something that would never have happened naturally in nature and, therefore, they are problematic. There are now 40,000 lawsuits pending. Eat organic. It's so important to your health.

Are you beginning to understand the magic of colors in fruits and veggies?

*Everyone with a chronic illness is so busy
looking for the magic pill. The magic is in
the colors of our fruits and vegetables.*

*Real fruits and veggies are the magic pill.
We have been looking in the wrong place.*

*The magic won't come from a phar-
maceutical. It comes from nature.*

Yellow

Yellow foods include:

Bananas
Garbanzo beans
Ginger
Golden kiwi
Grapefruit
Lemon
Pineapples
Plantains
Sweet corn
Yellow apples
Yellow beets
Yellow figs
Yellow lentils
Yellow pears
Yellow peppers
Yellow potatoes
Yellow potatoes
Yellow string beans
Yellow summer squash
Yellow tomatoes
Yellow watermelon
Yellow winter squash

Yellow fruits and vegetables also improve our immune function.

- Yellow Fruits and Vegetables Improve Immune Function.
- They are high in antioxidants like Vitamin C.
- They keep our teeth healthy.
- Heal cuts
- Help to absorb iron
- Prevent inflammation
- Improve circulation
- Have potassium
- Lowers cholesterol, lowers blood pressure
- Protect the skin from the sun and pollution
- Lemons act as an antacid and restore natural gastric function.
- Promote Eye Health
- Encourage alkaline balance
- Decrease the risk of some cancers
- Promote collagen formation and healthy joints
- Reduce the Risk of Heart Disease
- Promote collagen production protecting joints

Yellow is an amazing color. Now, let's talk about the amazing lemon.

I am so lucky; I have three Meyer's lemon trees in my backyard, and I admit I hoard them when they are in season. They grow especially large, and they aren't too tart or too sweet. They are loaded with juice. When I have lemons on my tree, I use lemon juice in all the water that I drink. Even though it is acidic, it turns alkaline in my tummy, and I am sure it is good for my health. My urologist just informed me that drinking lemon in my water also maintains the correct electrolyte balance in my body. I am anxiously waiting for my new batch now. They are growing, but currently a dark green, even though they have started acquiring size. I can't wait until they turn yellow and I can pick them again.

Why do I love lemons? Oh, let me count the ways:

- Lemons can be sweet, sour, and downright pucker-inducing.
- Lemons can be used in savory dishes and sweet treats.

- Lemons are antibacterial cleaning agents.
- Lemons are high in vitamin C and support heart health.
- Lemons reduce cancer risk.
- Lemons have small amounts of potassium, folate, and B-6 and iron.
- Lemons help aid digestion.
- Lemons have pectin, which is a soluble fiber that may help reduce total cholesterol.
- Lemon polyphenols also may improve insulin and leptin levels.
- Lemon juice is a powerful antimicrobial agent.
- Lemons prevent kidney stones.

Green

Green foods are associated with your heart and lungs and offer more health benefits.

These are the green fruits and veggies:

Artichokes
Arugula
Asparagus
Avocados
Broccoli
Brussel sprouts
Celery
Chayote squash
Chinese cabbage
Cucumbers
Endive
Fennel
Green apples

Green beans
Green cabbage
Green grapes
Green onion
Green pears
Honeydew
Leafy greens
Leeks
Lettuce
Limes
Okra
Peas
Snow peas
Soy (organic only)
Spinach
Sugar snap peas
Watercress
Zucchini

The best part of eating green veggies and fruits is that they are so alkaline. Cancer loves an acidic environment, so eating an alkaline diet is so important to stave off cancer.

- Green veggies are anti-carcinogenic and detoxifying.
- Green veggies create antioxidant activity.
- They help blood vessel expansion.
- They help the body with clotting.
- They are important for detoxification.
- They are important for metabolism.

"Leafy green vegetables are an important part of a healthy diet. They're packed with vitamins, minerals, and fiber but low in calories.

Eating a diet rich in leafy greens can offer numerous health benefits, including reduced risk of obesity, heart disease, high blood pressure, and mental decline."[15]

Broccoli, in the green family, has almost magical qualities. It's the stuff the heals and rebuilds the gut wall when it becomes "leaky." Pretty amazing stuff.

Aquamarine foods

Aquamarine foods (from the sea) Sea vegetables give you all 56 minerals and elements you need to survive. No other plant contains all 56.

Sea veggies are high in Iodine; you need some regularly, but do not overdo.

Sea Vegetables you should be eating:

Armani is brown kelp. Sweet, mild taste

Chlorella is anti-cancer, heavy metal and toxin removal, and mineral rich. It strengthens the liver function and removes poisons from the blood. It is the highest known source of chlorophyll and is loaded with protein.

Dulse is soft and has a chewy texture, is a reddish-brown color. Dulse is loaded with nutritional benefits and includes nutrients like beta-carotene, is it alkaline, loaded with vitamin C, many of the B vitamins, vitamin E, manganese, calcium, Iodine, potassium, iron, and zinc. Just a quarter of an ounce of dulse provides approximately 30% of the recommended daily allowance for iron. A single cup of dulse offers an incredible 4-6 grams of protein. Dulse makes a delicious snack at any time of the day.

Hijiki is packed with calcium and protein. On cooking, hijiki expands nearly four times and can be added to noodles or stir-fries with carrots onions and tofu. It has a strong flavor. This vegetable is rich in dietary fiber as well as essential minerals, including calcium, magnesium, and iron.

Kelp is an alga that grows in ocean water and is loaded with essential minerals, vitamins, and Iodine. High in folate, vitamin K, B-2, B-5, Iodine, magnesium, iron, copper, vitamin E, phosphorus, calcium, manganese, sodium, and zinc. Kelp is great in soups and stews. The versatility of kelp makes it easy to integrate into your diet. Kelp is excellent for keeping your digestive system and pancreas in top working condition.

Nori is mostly used for wrapping sushi. Also, Nori is delicious toasted. It is rich in beta-carotene, copper, manganese, potassium, phosphorus, folate, vitamin C, B-1, B-2, B-3, B-5, B-6, Iodine, vitamin E, iron, zinc, calcium, omega three and sodium. 28% protein

Sea Lettuce bears a strong resemblance to traditional lettuce, except that it possesses a strong seafood odor and taste. It easily crumbles into small tender pieces, which may be used in food preparations.

The gifts of Sea vegetables

- Main dietary source of Iodine
- Reduces risk of hyperlipidemia, coronary heart disease, and metabolic syndrome
- Sea vegetables support thyroid and balance thyroid function
- Protect your hormones, your metabolism, breathing, heart rate, nervous system, weight, body temperature, energy levels
- Sea vegetables can provide anti-aging benefits
- Cancer-fighting properties
- Sea veggies help improve mineral deficiencies
- Reduce the risk of hyperlipidemia, coronary heart disease, and metabolic syndrome
- Sea vegetables support thyroid and balance thyroid function

- Protect your hormones, your metabolism, breathing, heart rate, nervous system, weight, body temperature, and energy levels
- Sea vegetables can provide anti-aging benefits
- Cancer-fighting properties
- Sea veggies help improve mineral deficiencies
- They lower cholesterol
- They fight the effects of aging as well as chronic diseases.
- Sea vegetables represent Truth
- Improve hair, skin, and nails
- Excellent detox properties, removes toxins, heavy metals, and radioactive elements from the body
- Are rich in magnesium
- Reduce blood pressure

It is important that you get your Iodine from vegetables and not from Iodized salt.

Purple and blue

Purple and blue fruits and veggies are loaded with phytochemicals that are anti-inflammatory and boost our immune system.

Vegetables and fruits that fit into this color category include:

Black currants
Blackberries
Blueberries
Eggplant
Elderberries
Figs
Plums
Prunes
Purple asparagus

Purple cabbage
Purple carrots
Purple grapes
Purple peppers
Purple potatoes
Raisins

The benefits of this color are so important. I know that when I get a "flare" from my autoimmune disease, (which means that I gain 5 pounds overnight and am all puffy, but fortunately I no longer have the pain that used to come with a flare) I add resveratrol to my regime as it gives my body a boost, along with my curcumin and my quercetin to return to normal.

Dr. Tierona Low Dog, an Integrative MD who is also a Native American herbalist, often integrates information learned from her American Indian Grandmother. She says that studies have proven that Elderberry and Echinacea work together as well as Theraflu for the Flu or a cold. I always have these two items in my medicine box, along with resveratrol, curcumin, and quercetin. I prefer a natural approach, and for me, it works like a charm. If I am getting a cold or the Flu, I increase this color family on my plate so that I get the magic directly from the plant.

These are the other benefits from this color family:

- Blue and purple produce are anti-inflammatory (fights inflammation).
- They reduce inflammation.
- They may slow the onset of Alzheimer's.
- They can prevent blood clots.
- They are anti-viral.
- They protect the immune system.
- They protect cells from damage.
- They keep the gastrointestinal system healthy.
- They improve memory, cognition, and logic.
- Some purple and blue foods have resveratrol, which protects against Alzheimer's disease.
- They are rich in antioxidants.

- They are rich in phytonutrients reducing oxidative stress and chronic disease.
- They fight cancer and reduce the risk of cancer, they slow the progression of cancer, and they slow tumor growth.
- They act as an anticarcinogen in the digestive tract.
- They promote longevity.
- They help keep the eyes healthy, especially the retina.
- They improve calcium and mineral absorption.
- They are an excellent source of quercetin.
- Some blue and purple foods are high in Serotonin and Dopamine, which are the feel-good chemicals.
- They are often high in Vitamin C.
- Purple potatoes are high in Vitamin B-6.
- These colors are anti-diabetes.
- They are anti-aging.
- They promote youthful skin.

White and brown

The Gifts of White and Brown Fruits and Veggies and their importance to detoxification:

White and Brown Fruits and Vegetables Protect Against Certain Cancers, Keep Bones Strong, and Are A Heart-Healthy Choice

Bananas
Belgium endive
Cauliflower
Daikon radish
Fennel
Garlic

Ginger
Green onions
Jerusalem artichokes
Jicama
Mushrooms
Onions
Parsnips
Potatoes
Shallots
White cabbage
White nectarines
White peaches
White pears

This color group also have multiple gifts for the body:

- White and brown produce protects against cardiovascular disease.
- They reduce cholesterol.
- They can lower blood pressure.
- They can lower the risk of various heart ailments.
- Onions, garlic, jicama, shallots, and leeks are prebiotics. This one is so important. Most of us know by now how important healthy prebiotics are in the gut, but do you realize that they need to eat?

Prebiotics are the foods that feed our probiotics. Artichoke, Jerusalem artichokes, and chicory are also prebiotics.

- They are powerful antioxidants.
- They reduce inflammation.
- They help resist bone loss. Bone broth and these veggies are so much more effective to resist bone loss than dairy, which exacerbates the problem. Dairy is acidic, so your kidneys pull calcium from your bones to protect themselves. Eat white and brown veggies to improve your bone density.
- Garlic and onions have compounds that are important for the activity of enzymes that help remove toxins from your body. They are important to remove toxic metals, pesticides, unsafe additives from food products, and

even improve emotionally toxic experiences, relationships, and thoughts. I love this one since I have learned just how harmful toxic load is to the body. (A toxin is any substance that can adversely affect the function of cells in your body, causing fatigue, weight gain, skin problems, headaches, allergies, and depression.)

- They are a great source of dietary fiber.
- They reduce triglycerides. People commonly think that triglycerides are from fat. They are not; they are from sugar. And once triglycerides get high, they are stubborn to lower. Eat white veggies.
- They improve immune function.
- They fight infection, germs, and parasites.
- Allicin in garlic is antibacterial and anti-viral.
- They help protect against cancer.
- They reduce the risk of colon, breast, and prostate cancer.
- Garlic and onion may protect you from liver cancer.
- They balance our hormone system, reducing the risk of hormone-related cancers.
- Beta-glucan in mushrooms supports our white blood cells.

Note—People with allium allergy react negatively to onions, shallots, leeks, asparagus, and chives.

Antioxidants

List of the top antioxidant foods (and they come in all colors)

Allspice
Artichokes
Blueberries
Cilantro
Cinnamon
Clove

Coffee
Curly kale
Dark chocolate
Goji berries
Oregano
Pecans
Peppermint
Purple cabbage

The amazing benefits of these foods are:

- **Clove**—A 2010 study published in *Flavour and Fragrance Journal* found that clove is the best natural antioxidant thanks to its high levels of phenolic compounds. While often associated with the holidays, ground clove has a sweet-meets-savory flavor. You can use it in hummus, soups, and many other flavorful dishes.
- **Purple Cabbage**—This brightly colored veggie is the world's cheapest source of antioxidants per ounce—so stock up!
- **Curly Kale**—This increasingly popular cruciferous vegetable is one of the world's most nutrient-dense foods, and it contains a whopping serving of antioxidants including beta-carotene and vitamin C, plus vitamins K and B-6, as well as manganese, calcium, copper, potassium, and magnesium.
- **Artichokes**—According to the *Nutrition Journal* study, artichokes are among the top antioxidant-rich veggies. But don't just eat the hearts—the leaves contain a lot of the good stuff! If you've never cooked whole artichokes, it's easier than it appears. (And they are delicious.)
- **Oregano**—A great addition to plant-based pizza or almost any savory dish, oregano is big on taste and nutrient density. Research has found it to be a strong antioxidant and anti-carcinogenic. You can also easily grow it at home, along with other antioxidant-rich herbs, such as rosemary, thyme, and sage.
- **Peppermint**—Everyone's favorite minty herb is a powerful antioxidant. It's packed with manganese; copper; vitamins A, B-6, C, E, and K; beta-carotene; folate; riboflavin; and more. Fresh peppermint is great steeped into a fragrant tea! Just crush the leaves and add hot water.

- **Allspice**—This versatile spice contains vitamin A, vitamin C, eugenol, quercetin, and tannins, all combined to make it a strong addition to your diet. You can use allspice in sweet dishes. And for extra flavor, try adding it to stews, curries, and soups.
- **Cinnamon**—Cinnamon has countless applications in cooking, and it's full of polyphenols. In a 2005 study published in the *Journal of Agricultural and Food Chemistry*, cinnamon topped a list of 26 spices for its high antioxidant properties.
- **Cilantro**—This love-it-or-hate-it herb is big on the flavonoid quercetin, as well as iron, magnesium, and manganese. If you like cilantro, you may find it to be a delicious addition to salads, summer rolls, or guacamole.
- **Blueberries**—These tasty berries are among the most powerful antioxidants out there. A 2012 study published in the *Journal of Zhejiang University SCIENCE* found that blueberries packed the strongest antioxidant punch when compared with blackberries and strawberries. They've also been shown to fight cancer, help with weight loss, aid in digestion, and protect your brain and heart. *If you can, choose wild blueberries (often found in the frozen section) sometimes because they have nearly double the antioxidant content*. Frozen Blueberries have more antioxidants than fresh fruit! Be sure to avoid any with added sugar though, as *dried fruit has a high sugar content already*. Look for organic wild blueberries.
- **Dark Chocolate**—When it comes to chocolate, the higher the percentage of cocoa present in the product, the better. Dark chocolate has a wealth of antioxidant compounds, including polyphenols, flavonols, and catechins. A 2011 study published in the study *Chemistry Central Journal* found that *dark chocolate had more antioxidant capacity than any of the superfruits, including blueberries and acai berries*.
- I also just found some 70% cocoa sweetened with stevia and have it on order to try from Pascha. (It's soy-free)
- Lily's makes vegan, fair trade, sugar-free dark chocolates that are remarkably delicious.
- **Pecans**—A 2011 study published in *The Journal of Nutrition* concluded that this tree nut's unique mix of antioxidants (including one form of vitamin E called gamma-tocopherols) might help prevent heart disease.

After participants ate pecans, the unhealthy oxidation of LDL (bad) cholesterol in their blood decreased by as much as 33%. Eat a handful as an afternoon pick-me-up.

- **Goji Berries**—A staple of traditional Chinese medicine for centuries, these little red berries have only recently become more mainstream. They are loaded with antioxidants. According to a 2008 study published in the *Journal of Alternative and Complementary Medicine*, the benefits of goji berries include "increased ratings for energy levels, athletic performance, quality of sleep, ease of awakening, ability to focus on activities, mental acuity, calmness, feelings of health, contentment and happiness, and significantly reduced fatigue and stress." *Goji berries can be pricey, and I find it arguable whether they're better for you than less exotic options, like strawberries or blueberries. But there's little doubt they're rich in antioxidants.*

- **Coffee**—This popular beverage turns out to have loads of antioxidants. In fact, coffee is *the #1 source of antioxidants in the American diet*—by a wide margin. Coffee is a very dirty crop, so be sure to buy and drink it organic.

How do you take the goodness that comes from the colors of the plants and maximize their benefit in your body?

Choose complexity; every day, eat as many colors as possible. Move synergistically through the spectrum of health. The combination of colors in your daily meals will reward you with good health. I suggest you eat three different veggies each night as a minimum.

Eat half your veggies raw and half your veggies lightly cooked. Steaming veggies for 2-3 minutes, many release their gifts to a form easily utilized by the body. Three-quarters of your daily food should be plants, preferably organic.

Roasting vegetables brings out their best flavor. Shake in a bag with a little ghee, organic garlic, and organic onion powder and pepper (I used Primal Palate Steak mix, yum) spread out on a baking sheet (I use parchment paper underneath) and cook at 400 until roasted. Leave them slightly crunchy.

Make good partnerships with your food using healing spices in your cooking. As an example, the combination of turmeric, black pepper, and olive oil releases all its pain-reducing healing properties. Spices also make your food infinitely more interesting

Add ginger when stir-frying for its healing and pain-reducing properties. I also love to make ginger tea. Just cut off a slice and let it brew in hot water. Add a little raw stevia, and it's delicious.

Adding rosemary or thyme protects you from cancer.

Cinnamon reduces blood sugar.

Add parsley, which is exceptionally high in lutein, and great for eyesight. When I was a little girl, I already had tons of allergies. (I believe now that they were actually sensitivities.) I couldn't eat the cookies and snacks that other children could eat, so my Mother would give me a handful of parsley to munch on. To this day, I love parsley. I will sit in a restaurant and ask permission to eat the parsley off everyone's plate. I love, love, love it.

Avocado not only has excellent oils for the body but is a powerhouse for fiber and lycopene, which encourages heart health.

Eat foods high in quercetin (onions, berries, apples, and capers) for its anti-inflammatory characteristics healing the kidneys, the gut, the liver, and reducing allergies. Remember, quercetin is also very good for the brain.

The key is to use them all and to mix them together for optimal health.

Mix it up, find new foods, and eat them often.

Finally, eat plants several times a day. Add a handful of spinach and onion to your morning eggs. Add berries (frozen or fresh) to your morning organic oatmeal. Make colorful salads for lunch. Use fruit as your afternoon snack. Find as many ways as possible to incorporate multiple colors of fruits and veggies in your daily food plan.

Your body will celebrate.

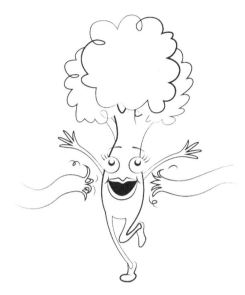

Chapter 4

"Use This/Not That" Ingredient Guide to Make Any Recipe Healthy

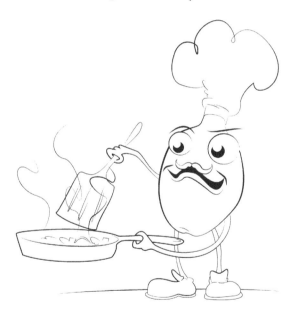

THE BIG TAKEAWAYS ON "USE THIS NOT THAT" INGREDIENT GUIDE:[16]

- *If you have pain, you should have yourself tested for sensitivities. I recommend Meridian Valley in Seattle if your MD will not order the test from Genova Labs. You don't need an MD to order from Meridian Valley, you can order yourself. You get a 1-hour consultation with their MD when you get your results.*

- *Cook, it's the only way to control what you are putting into your body.*

- *Whenever possible, substitute healthier ingredients for ingredients that are less healthy.*

- *Using this guide, you can swap out ingredients and make any recipe healthier. This is what I use to cook.*

- *Remember, you must cook, but it doesn't need to be complicated. Roasted veggies are delicious and about as easy to make as it comes.*

- *Your evening meal should include a protein source, three different colors of veggies, and a carb. If you keep quality ingredients on hand, it becomes easier to cook each night.*

There are so many hidden toxins in our food; it is important to cook most of what we are going to eat so that we can control what we are putting into our bodies.

1   I personally only buy organic. If you think that is too expensive, you at least need to follow the guidelines published every year by EWG, for the dirty dozen and the clean 15. The dirty dozen are the vegetables and fruits with the most toxins on them. If you want to learn about what is being sprayed on our food that is poisoning your body, buy my first book. Avoid all GMOs and look for the non-GMO label. For a good explanation of what GMO is, refer to my first book.[17]

2   I avoid using processed foods loaded with chemicals and avoid things like canned soup because of the ingredients and the BPA in the cans. If you can't pronounce an ingredient or if you don't know what it is, like

"natural flavors," pass. They are synthetic chemicals that your body cannot use. Often, they are one of 40 names for MSG.

3   Avoid Carmel color. It is made from a secretion from a beaver's butt. Careful, caramel color is in broths and soups, and it's really not good for you, so read labels carefully.

4   Avoid carrageenan. It is a possible carcinogen. (Look for it in everything. It's in personal care products like toothpaste, food, milk, pet food, etc.)

5   By cooking, you ensure the maximum number of nutrients to fuel your body and, you control what is going into your body.

6   Next, I should share that I have sensitivities to 15 different foods, so I have become very inventive in the kitchen to make old favorites. As a result, I am a fast order cook. And I swap out a lot of ingredients. I love to eat. I cook unusual but yummy food.

If you want to be checked for sensitivities, there is now an at-home test that you can order from Meridian Valley Labs. (855 405 TEST) You do not need a doctor to order it for you. You prick your finger and send it in, and then get the results. Learning which foods, I was sensitive to allowed me to eliminate a chunk of my pain from autoimmune disease. For an explanation of sensitivity vs. an allergy, refer to my book, **It Feels Good to Feel Good, Learn to Eliminate Toxins, Reduce Inflammation, and Feel Great Again**.[18]

So, let's talk about how I approach cooking.

1   It starts with having great ingredients on hand. I keep the dry goods below in my pantry so that they are always on hand to use.

2   I always have fresh farmers market vegetables and fruits on hand.

3   My freezer has grass-fed/ grass-finished beef in a variety of different cuts, wild-caught fish, mostly salmon, lamb, and heritage pastured pork in a couple of different cuts. Chicken is a sensitivity for me now, but if I could eat it, I would have a level 4 or 5 chicken[19,20] frozen in my freezer. Since I cannot eat chicken, I often have a turkey breast and thighs in my freezer instead.

4   One of the first things I do in the morning is to take the meat out of the freezer that I plan to cook for our evening meal.

I then survey the veggies I have on hand to make a salad with that are in my fridge and what other veggies I have to complete my meal.

If I need a recipe, I have listed the cookbooks that I frequent at the end of this chapter. What I often do is search for a Paleo recipe for what I want to cook right on the internet. I eat Paleo (or what Dr. Hyman calls "Pegan," lower meat quantity), and Paleo recipes are clean and will most often call for the ingredients that I keep on hand.

If I can't find what I am looking for, I Google for a regular recipe and then convert it to healthy using the substitutions below.

DAIRY FREE CREAM SAUCE

I cannot have dairy, it's kryptonite to me, so if I want a cream sauce, depending on what dish I am using it in, I will prepare soaked cashew nuts, (preferably overnight) and/or steamed cauliflower. Or I would use almond cream instead of dairy cream. (It is harder to find. It's made by Califia). These ingredients all get a spin in my Vitamix. I then add sea salt and the appropriate seasonings, and I always add ghee to add richness.

I have even made dishes like Swedish meatballs and clam chowder using my cauliflower and cashew cream sauce (with mushrooms and onions, garlic, and almond cream from Califia).

Instead of dairy milk, I use Califia Almond milk and cream, or SO Organic Cashew and Almond milk in the new biodegradable bottle or MALK. You can also make your own.

SOUR CREAM and YOGURT

I avoid both from cows since it is a major sensitivity for me. There are some wonderful yogurts available now made with almond milk or cashew milk. Kite Hill makes regular and Greek-style almond yogurt. Kite Hill also just introduced almond sour cream, brilliant. I use these to replace sour cream.

RANCH DRESSING

Ranch dressing is something that I missed when I went dairy-free. I found a recipe by Danielle Walker (one of my favorite recipe writers of all time listed below) for a ranch dressing with chicken wings. I don't make the chicken wings, but I make this ranch dressing all the time, and I love it. It has all the flavor of the regular ranch dressing without the dairy. It's probably the salad dressing that we utilize the most. http://bit.ly/dwalkerranchdressing

We buy Primal kitchen Thousand Island dressing with avocado oil, as well. I am discovering that I love all the Primal Kitchen salad dressings. (As of this writing, there are now many Primal Kitchen salad dressings that we enjoy, including a vegan ranch.) We also use Soy-Free Follow Your Heart Mayo and make Thousand Island dressing. We use a lot of Braggs Apple Cider Vinegar with the mother and olive oil for salads. I have four lemon trees, and my lemons are huge and juicy, so I love it when they are in season. Make sure you use quality olive oil that has an olive color. (Make sure it is either from California where it is regulated to actually be olive oil in the bottle or use European olive oil that has a certification on the bottle that it IS olive oil.)

CONDIMENTS

We use **Primal Kitchen organic unsweetened BBQ Sauce**, and their **ketchup** and **mustard**. **Follow Your Heart Soy Free Mayo**, and my latest find is **No Soy (Soy Fee) Soy** sauce and **Teriyaki Sauce** by Ocean's Halo. It's not as good as soy sauce, but it's also not GMO or soy, so it's close, and I am happy. (Soy is one of my sensitivities, and 95% of soy is GMO)

BUTTER AND MARGARINE

Since I can't use butter, I use ghee in its place. Ghee is organic clarified butter, which means the milk solids that I am sensitive to are removed. It adds the taste of butter without the downside. Ghee is especially good for your body if you have an autoimmune disease. Ghee has SCFA butyrate. Virgin coconut oil (anti-candida) is also a good choice. I don't care for the smell and taste of coconut, so I use ghee.

If canola oil is on the ingredient list or vegetable oil (corn, soy, soybean, cotton-seed, sugar beet oils), I will substitute olive oil, coconut oil, ghee, or avocado oil. I would never use margarine. I never liked the taste, and it is pure chemicals and GMO oils.

We eat at a couple of farm-to-table restaurants in Sedona that use rice bran oil. Yummy and not GMO. Good for us as well.

If you CAN use butter, please use organic butter so that you aren't getting a healthy dose of toxins or artificial hormones from the butter. Ideally, use raw organic milk butter. There are things in raw milk that work together, synergistically, for your body's health.

TOMATO PRODUCTS

I want organic since tomatoes are often GMO now. They are also a dirty crop. And, because of how acidic tomatoes are, I only buy tomato products in glass. I use organic Jovial Tomatoes in jars and their crushed tomatoes. Organic tomato paste is also available in a jar. I do still cheat and use RAO's spaghetti sauce, it is not organic, but I think it has a superior taste to other spaghetti sauces. We also use RAO's pizza sauce. I keep my toxic load so low that this one slip, I think, is ok.

PIZZA

So, what do we use as a crust to make pizza?

Cappello's Naked Pizza Crust

We bought a steel plate that goes into our oven 1 hour before we are ready to make our pizza so that it gets good and hot. You can buy one on Amazon, and it gets the crust to pizza texture. Ceramic stones are also available.

There has been a lot of spiel about cauliflower pizza crusts, and you would think I would love that, right? Well, read the ingredients on the box. There are other ingredients in many of these that I don't want to eat, and Cappello's crust keeps changing ingredients, but they are always clean ingredients that are good for me. So, I stick with them.

Reminder: always read your label, no matter who recommends something. Ingredients change. (And what one person thinks is healthy might not meet your criteria).

CHEESE

Since I found out I am dairy sensitive, cheese is the #1 thing that I miss. I have tried several times to see if I have outgrown the sensitivity, and I always react, so it's just not worth how I blow up and get pain when I try it again.

Fortunately, over time, there are better and better vegan cheeses available.

Kite Hill has a pretty good ricotta cheese. (As does Dr. Weil at his True Food Restaurants, but they don't sell theirs, they only serve it. They say it is just almonds and water. I haven't tried to make it.) Kite Hill also makes good cream cheeses. Recently we found Miyoko makes a great chive cream cheese that is delicious with lox.

My new favorites are VIOLIFE cheeses. They have a Provolone that is quite yummy and a Parmesan cheese. I also use their Feta, mozzarella, and cheddar. (Whole Foods)

I like the rounds of Miyoko vegan cheese. I made scalloped potatoes and ham with their cheddar round. I use Parmela Creamery nut cheeses, especially in salads.

RICE, PASTA, AND POTATOES

CAULIFLOWER

I will often make cauliflower rice instead of a carb white or brown rice. Cauliflower takes on whatever flavor you want. I have made cauliflower Italian, Greek, Moroccan, and I made paella with it with saffron and even made it with apples, garlic and onions once.

For Italian, I added Italian seasoning. (Primal Palate) I then added sundried tomato, and onion, celery, (If you can have it, parmesan cheese otherwise the VioLife parmesan is a good substitution).

For Greek, I added a spice mix that was Greek with oregano (Primal Palate), and then sundried tomatoes, Greek olives, red pepper, (if you can have it, feta cheese, otherwise the VioLife is a good substitution)

For Moroccan, I add cumin and cinnamon, let it soak in the hot ghee that I add to the pan to bring out its aroma, and then garlic and onion. Raisins, dried apricots, and dried cherries top it off, and then I roast slivers of almonds right in the ghee in the pan. (My husband will make harissa sauce with 2/3 ground cayenne pepper and 1/3 cumin, and then he adds enough water to make a thick sauce. I am a hot spice wuss, so this is way too hot for me.

MASHED CAULIFLOWER

Cauliflower also is fantastic mashed instead of potatoes and loaded with wonderful nutrients. I had one guest tell me my mashed cauliflower was bar-none the best mashed potatoes they had ever eaten. I make it with almond milk and ghee in my Vitamix. (not too moist, fluffy like potatoes.)

PASTA, RICE, AND GRAINS

I thought I was sensitive to gluten until I went to Italy on my honeymoon. Ends up, I am only sensitive to non-organic pasta and bread. It's the Glyphosate in conventional wheat. I still limit how much I eat. The functional medicine community thinks you should avoid gluten, no matter what.

ONLY EAT ORGANIC pasta if you choose to eat wheat pasta. Before the wheat harvest, the conventional wheat is drowned in glyphosate (Roundup), and none of that gets washed off before it gets made into processed foods, wheat products, pasta, bread, etc. Since we now know that Roundup causes cancer (as of the end of 2019, they have lost three lawsuits), you should avoid anything with Roundup on it at all costs.

I also avoid white rice and white rice products because of the way they grow white rice, and it is loaded with arsenic. Brown rice has even more arsenic.

I use Lundberg rice mixes because of their growing methods. Basmati rice from California is the lowest in arsenic. All California rice appears to be less toxic. (Texas rice is the highest.)

We like quinoa as a side dish. It's a healthy grain and yummy with ghee and mushrooms and veggies mixed in.

Spaghetti Squash is a wonderful substitution for whole wheat pasta.

Spiralized zucchini is another wonderful substitution for whole wheat pasta.

POTATOES

In the beginning, when I first got sick, I avoided potatoes. They are in the night-shade family, to which many people are sensitive. Nightshades, however, do not happen to be a problem for me. We ONLY eat organic potatoes. Make sure you eat the skins, which is where most of the nutrition is. There are 35 pesticides used on conventionally grown potatoes.[21]

Human Health Effects of a conventional potato:[22]

6	—	Known or Probable Carcinogens
12	—	Suspected Hormone Disruptors
7	—	Neurotoxins
6	—	Developmental or Reproductive Toxins

Environmental Effects:

9	—	Honeybee Toxins—(they kill our bees. No bees, no pollination, no crops)

These are not an everyday item in my diet.

If I mash them, I mash them with the skin and ghee and almond milk.

We do eat sweet potatoes more often. They have tons of nutrition packed in them and are delicious baked or mashed.

On a rare occasion, we eat potato chips. Only organic, only in oil that I approve like ghee or avocado.

SUGAR AND OTHER SWEETENERS

Instead of sugar or fake sugar, I cut the sweet way down, probably in half and use honey, maple syrup, or coconut sugar. They are still sugar but contain trace elements that are healthy. Things taste better when they are less sweet, and sugar is toxic. My preferred natural sweetener is coconut sugar because it is low glycemic. It also has the rich taste of brown sugar.

Sometimes I use applesauce for part of the sweet, like in cakes. I have also used bananas to lower the sweet. Dates are also an excellent sweetener, and I use those in recipes. There is an entire chapter about the dangers of sugar and how addictive it is in my first book.[23]

- Fake sugars are just that, fake. They are poisons. Pink and blue packets are neurotoxins. The yellow packet kills your good gut bacteria. Avoid them. I only use Stevia, but make sure it is just Stevia, and that it doesn't have other ingredients added in (like dextrose. Dextrose is the name of a simple sugar chemically identical to glucose (blood sugar) that is made from corn (BT Toxin)).
- I recently read that Stevia in alcohol also has downsides for your health because of what they do to get Stevia out of the leaf. We now use green stevia leaf that has been powdered by Mayan. It doesn't dissolve the same way but otherwise works well.

I don't like to cook with Stevia; I don't like the taste. I don't often bake, again, that is not something we indulge in on an everyday basis. Went I do bake, I use honey, maple syrup or coconut sugar.

Avoid Agave. It is harder on the liver than any of the sugars. Hard to believe something is harder on the body, but Agave is.

I don't use any of the alcohol sweeteners. **Erythritol** goes right through me, so I avoid it. The other sugar alcohols are no better. They are mostly made from GMO corn, so read the labels, and I recommend avoiding them all as well. Sorbitol is a baby laxative, so no wonder my body responds the way that it does. Sugar alcohols are in lots of products, so be aware of what you are eating when you read the label.

I have a friend that makes delicious baked goods using monk fruit. Make sure that dextrose is not one of the ingredients. Monk fruit is a great choice again because it is low glycemic. Most Monk Fruit sweeteners have the Erythritol in them. Julian Bakery[24] makes one that is just monk fruit.

WHIPPED CREAM

For whipping cream, I use coconut cream. Careful to buy it in BPA free cans. Get them really cold in the refrigerator. Then it whips just like dairy cream. Add a little stevia (all Stevia, no other added ingredients) and add a little real organic vanilla, and it is yummy.

CHOCOLATE AND COCOA

I use organic cocoa. And I use 70% dark chocolate morsels. (or 69%) (Real Life, also soy-free) We do have a piece of chocolate at night, soy-free, from Theo. Make sure all your chocolate is 70% (or close) and that it doesn't have soy lecithin (GMOs).

TEA AND COFFEE

I buy Yogi, Numi, and Traditional Medicinals tea in paper bags. Those cute little triangular bags are plastic, so they are poison in hot water. The teas I recommend are also organic and washed. If I am drinking coffee, I drink only organic coffee. If I am struggling with adrenal issues and chronic fatigue, I skip the coffee. My body doesn't need additional stimulation.

If I am feeling good, then my coffee of choice is organic Mayorga Café Cubano. It's a dark roast organic coffee with a deep rich flavor.

SPICES

I use organic spices and seasonings from Primal Palate. For Italian, I use Amore. I add their garlic and onion powder to everything. I love their barbeque spice rub, and my secret ingredient when I cook is the steak seasoning blend. I also use their organic cinnamon and their cloves and nutmeg. For vanilla, I use Simply Organics. They also do nice organic blends.

BONE BROTH

Bone broth is good for us. I am not much inclined to make my own and often buy frozen bone broth that is grass-fed grass-finished at one of my organic grocers.

I always have boxed beef bone broth in my pantry. Kettle and Fire is a great brand, but I am a member of Thrive Market, and I prefer their in-house brand. I also always have their turkey bone broth on hand. I will often decide to make soup when I have lots of good veggies in my fridge. I also buy turkey (on the bone) to bake with the intention of using the leftovers to make turkey soup. I use beef (grass-fed grass-finished) in sauces, in my veggie soups where I steam a veggie and then give it a whirl in my Vitamix I always add bone broth, and sometimes I use it to steam my veggies. There are tons of frozen bone broths available. I must be careful that they didn't include chicken feet when making it, even beef broth. They want its collagen. As noted previously, I react to the chicken.

MEATS

For meat, I use grass-fed grass-finished beef, pastured heritage pork, and pastured poultry. All sheep eat grass, so you are safe with lamb. We only eat wild fish. Bison like grass, so they are also a great choice. If you can't get good meat in the winter, try Wellness Meat in Missouri. If you buy a certain amount, they ship free. We buy our meat, if possible, from our rancher in Sedona. He too has autoimmune disease and is careful of what he feeds his herd year-round. (And his beef is delicious.)

EGGS

I use pastured eggs. (not cage-free). We do buy pastured eggs on occasion at farmer's markets. Otherwise, we use Vital Farms organic eggs. You want eggs from chickens that are outdoors except when they need protection from the weather, and the chickens need to eat their natural diet of grasses, berries, and insects. (The insects make them tasty.)

FLOURS

For flours, depending on what I am making, I would use almond flours for baked goods and cookies, or cassava flour for pie crusts. Often a mixture of coconut flours with almond flours gets the best results in baked goods. Danielle Walker recipes call for this. I like Honeyville blanched almond flour because of how fine it is, and I like the texture of how it bakes. I use almond flour for killer scones and cupcakes etc.

I use organic all-purpose flour from Bobs Mills for dredging and then sautéing fish, and I add my Primal Palate garlic, onion, and steak seasoning to make it interesting.

I use Trader Joe's aluminum-free baking powder and Bob's baking soda.

WAFFLES AND PANCAKES

I do make pancakes and waffles with almond flour. I also use the Simple Mills Pancake and Waffle mix, which is almond flour and clean ingredients. I make my own syrup using frozen organic berries, ghee, and a touch of maple syrup. Organic peaches also work. By using frozen berries, I cut the sugar way, way down, and yet keep the yummy factor.

SHORTENING

My mother always used CRISCO. It's now deadly with its ingredients, and it is GMO soy. I use Nutiva Organic Vegan Superfood Shortening instead.

OLIVE OIL

If the recipe calls for olive oil, I make sure it is either Californian or a certified Italian or Spanish oil that declares it is 100% olive oil. The mafia has gotten involved in the olive oil industry and is cutting it with less expensive oils. If it says California on the bottle, the olive oil is olive oil. There is a law on the books here that it must be 100% olive oil to say Californian. Remember, olive oils get rancid quickly, so store it in a dark-colored bottle in a dark place. They have a shelf life of about two years. Smell your olive oil before using it. You can smell it if it has gone rancid.

HOW I COOK

I take a recipe and go down the ingredient list and use the healthiest substitution possible. I can convert any recipe to a healthier version. I am not Julia Child, but I am a foodie, as is my hubby, so I make delicious, simple food.

Remember, it is important that you cook, but it doesn't need to be complicated. Roasted veggies are delicious and about as easy to make as it comes.

A balanced evening meal would consist of a high-quality protein source, at least three different veggies in different colors, and a carb source. Three-quarters of your plate should be veggies.

My favorite cookbooks are

- Danielle Walker: "**Against All Grain**" series.
- Carrie Vitt: "**Deliciously Organic**" series
- Melissa Joulwan: "The Well Fed Blog and Cookbooks"
- Michele Tam: "**NomNom Paleo**" series
- Debbie Barbiero is a health coach that teaches cooking, and I enjoy her cookbooks. Some of her cookbooks are available on Amazon. Others can be purchased directly from her by calling 203-929-9414 or email debshealthyplate@gmail.com
- Mark Hyman, MD's cookbook "Food: What the Heck Should I Cook?: More than 100 Delicious Recipes--Pegan, Vegan, Paleo, Gluten-free, Dairy-free, and More--For Lifelong Health." (NEW) Many of his friends have contributed recipes, and I know they will be healthy to make.
- They all have recipes for normal cooks that are delicious, easy to follow, not complicated, and relatively quick.

I am planning to put out my cookbook later this year to encourage everyone to cook using all the colors of the rainbow. I am a funny cook, since I cook around 15 sensitivities, and I read a recipe on the computer in my office and go to the kitchen and make it. But I think it's important to entice you to eat all the colors, so I plan to do my cookbook using normal preparation methods. *smile* I have found superfood powders in intense colors that will be a joy to cook with to wow you. My cookbook will be called "It Feels Good to Eat the Rainbow, Recipes to Feel Great."

Chapter 5

How to afford high-quality food on a budget, and why it's important

BUY ORGANIC	CAN BUY CONVENTIONAL
Dirty Dozen	**Clean 15**
1. Strawberries	1. Avocados
2. Spinach	2. Sweet corn
3. Kale	3. Pineapple
4. Nectarines	4. Onions
5. Apples	5. Papaya
6. Grapes	6. Sweet Peas (Frozen)
7. Peaches	7. Eggplant
8. Cherries	8. Asparagus
9. Pears	9. Cauliflower
10. Tomatoes	10. Cantaloupes
11. Celery	11. Broccoli
12. Potatoes	12. Mushrooms
	13. Cabbage
	14. Honeydew Melon
	15. Kiwi

It Feels Good To Feel Good

@ EWG 2020

Avoid the Dirty Dozen and GMOs

Food is fuel for the body. I think we forget this when we eat. If it is a good fuel, it gives us energy, make us clear-headed, and it makes us happy. If it is high-quality food, it makes our bodies feel good, and our bodies will sing.[25]

Good fuel tastes good. There is no deprivation in eating good food. Good food makes your body feel great, so it is well worth being the food that you eat. Good Food consists of whole foods without chemicals.

But there is a lot of bad food that also tastes good. Just because food tastes good, doesn't mean that it is good for your body. Bad food gives us bloating, drops in energy, fuzzy thinking, and has addictive ingredients in it that make us crave more of it. Bad food consists of synthetic ingredients that give our bodies no nutrients to function on, many of which are also harmful. I recently heard this referred to as "nutricide." Often bad food is loaded with added sugar, which is highly addictive and very harmful to our bodies. Bad food is also loaded with MSG, which now is in food under 39 different names. MSG is a neurotoxin. I have a theory that if I can't pronounce it, I don't buy it. And, if I don't know what the ingredient is, my body won't either and won't be able to utilize it, so I also don't buy it. This way, I avoid MSG in my food no matter what name they are calling it today. This way, I avoid all the fake ingredients.

If you have a child, this is even more important. If we want to safeguard our children to grow up in healthy bodies, we need to feed them real live food loaded with nutrients, and that doesn't come with a healthy dose of toxins. Most chronic conditions start in childhood, and these conditions are exacerbated by bad food, nutrient deficiencies, and toxic overload. Eliminating fake synthetic ingredients is the path to raise healthy, happy, and smart children. Feed them what will serve their bodies and their brains well.

If you have a chronic condition, it can also be this simple. The body wants to heal, but you must give it the nutrients that it needs and is able to use to bring us back to wellness. There is no magic pill that Abracadabra will return you to good health. Eat real live organic food, preferably from a farm as close to you as possible, and eat in season, and that includes all the available colors of fruits and vegetables. Eating real, live, organic food CAN bring you back to relative health. Why is it important to eat from a source close to you? Because then it has maximum nutrients to help your body function. It may not eliminate your chronic condition but will allow your body to function at an optimal level, and it will support your health. (The further the food is from the harvest; the more flavor and nutrients are lost.) If you don't have that available to you all year where you live, eat organic from further away areas, or eat organic frozen veggies and fruits.

If you are well, this will help to keep you well because you are feeding your body the nutrients that it needs, without the healthy dose of toxins that long term will make your body sick.

I read once, 25 years ago, that if I was overweight, which I was, it was because I was starving my body. At the time, this statement confused me. Now I "get" it. I was starving my body of the nutrients that my body needed to heal and remain healthy. As a result, my body kept craving MORE, to try and get the nourishment it was lacking from what I was putting into my body.

> *"Medicine is not Health Care. Food Is Health Care.*
> *Medicine is Sick Care.*
> *It is time we see it for what it is."*
>
> UNKNOWN[26]

Food is health care. You cannot rely on medicine to make you well. Use food so that you don't go down that chute in the first place.

It makes sense that you should pay more for organic, high-quality food. You pay more for a Cadillac or a Mercedes, and you pay it because you know you are getting more for your money. And yet, when we are buying food, we seem to think that good food is not worth the price, even though good food is one of the, if not THE one thing, that is important to keep our body and the bodies of our families in good health. Good food is an investment in good health, an unspoiled environment, fair treatment for animals, and tasty eating.

I am asking that you reframe how you think about high-quality organic food. It is one of the best investments you can make with your money. And in the long run, it will save you money because it will save you medical bills.

The reality is that poor quality food, conventionally grown food, is subsidized by our government. It makes no sense to me that our tax dollars go to growing food with pesticides and herbicides that are not respectful to our livestock, and that is destroying our environment. One of the reasons real healthy food costs more is because it is not government-subsidized like poor quality food is. We won't change that, but we should be aware of it. The government does not regulate conventional farming practices, many of which are disgusting right on the surface, so there is no surprise that conventional food is less healthy. Still, it costs less because our government gives conventional operations lots of money to keep the costs low to grow unhealthy food.

Our government heavily subsidizes industrial agriculture, making its products artificially cheap.

On the other hand, the government is very involved in regulating organic food. Those farmers and ranchers jump through continual hoops to ensure that their food is healthy. Our government is ensuring that healthy food practices are more expensive than unhealthy food practices. On the bright side, government regulations ensure that organic foods meet a higher standard than conventional foods and that they are what they say they are.

You can afford high-quality food if it is important to you. Ideally, I want you to cook 90% of your food. If you think real live food costs too much, it is too hard and takes too long, and you are relying on "convenience" foods, these "inexpensive convenience foods" will not be so convenient when they make you and your family ill. In the beginning, it takes more planning to eat real food, but in the long run, it has been proven that it is not more expensive,[27] and it doesn't need to take long to make. We are simply a society that has gotten into bad habits, and we are thinking "convenience" first out of habit. And convenience equates in our minds to "out of a box." "frozen with multiple ingredients," from a fast-food restaurant, or out at a regular restaurant where we do not usually know what goes into the food.

Could we reframe that to making a meal from real live food in under 30 minutes?

So, where do we start? I think the most important place to start is to look at where you are spending your food dollars now, and whether you could change some of that to save money?

1   Are you stopping often to buy coffee in the morning? Add up how much you are spending a week and save that money for quality food.

I now have a Melita[28] coffee pot, I boil filtered tap water and use organic coffee to make my morning joe. The pot and cone are only $12.99 on Amazon (2020), and since I am not paying over $4 for my cup at my local coffee chain, it pays for itself quickly. You only need to purchase inexpensive brown unbleached paper filters. I love a robust, dark coffee, and it has taken me some time to find an organic brand that I love. (Coffee is sprayed with tons of chemicals when it is conventionally grown, so this way I also get to enjoy my morning cup without the bonus of nasty herbicides and pesticides in my drink) I have settled on Mayorga Café Cubano coffee, and they run some great sales, so sign up for their mailing list. (He started growing organic coffee to help the communities that grow coffee too. The toxins sprayed on conventional coffee were making everyone in these communities ill. So now he grows organic coffee in these villages. They are healthier; we are healthier; the earth is healthier. Win-Win Win) I love, love, love the taste of his coffee. A rich dark brew. I drink Cubano.

I own a stainless-steel carafe[29] that keeps my coffee super-hot. So hot, that I leave the carafe open for several minutes before I put the lid on and take in in my bag. Since I no longer buy coffee on my way to work, the plastic from the store-bought coffee is also not leeching chemicals into my coffee. And the paper cups that hold the coffee have wax that has their own issues in my body.

2   How often are you going out for lunch during the week? Save that money and take your lunch from home. I know you want to eat with friends, take your lunch with you and order iced tea and still eat with your co-workers. It might feel a little awkward in the beginning, but you

are doing this for your health. Your friends will understand, and in most cases, the restaurant won't object. I do this all the time. I refuse to eat the SAD (Standard American Diet) because it made me sick, and I am not going there again.

By taking your lunch with you, you are also ensuring that you are feeding your body quality food that is organic and loaded with nutrients. By making your food, you are controlling what you are putting into your mouth and your body.

3   How often are you meeting friends and going out for dinner at night? Eating out costs more money than cooking at home. How about starting a supper club, and meeting at each other's homes and eating in community that way?

Have you heard of the 6 degrees of separation? Well, there is a ripple effect of 3 degrees of separation because our immediate community impacts our lifestyle. Whether it is obesity, smoking, alcohol abuse, or whether it is happiness, love, and success, people 3 degrees away from you impact your emotions and habits. People within 3 degrees of separation impact your health. Foster relationships that support your goal of being healthy.

Invite friends into your supper club based on how committed they are to healthy eating. If you are all committed to healthy eating, cooking for each other will bond you all together closer and support your efforts to eat well and feed your body what it needs without giving up the joy of community. It makes getting together fun.

If they are not committed to eating healthy and still want to be in the in-crowd, *smile*, then yes still have them come, and have them bring their own food. You bring healthy food and stick to it.

I will discuss how to eat in community with others who are not as committed to health later in this book in Chapters (7 & 8). For now, be the influencer that encourages others in your immediate social circle to support healthy eating habits.

Having a supper club also lowers the cost of drinking alcohol. How much does a single glass of wine cost when you go out? How could you better use those funds? For the same cost or less, rather than buying and sharing a bottle of wine in a restaurant, now you can drink a fine bottle of organic wine. Grapes are another dirtiest crop, so this way, you enjoy your wine without the nasty toxins. You can also save money by not drinking out. I am not suggesting that you never drink; I am just suggesting that you find a way to save part of that money to purchase healthier food.

4   Let's talk about snacks. And let's start with why you want them in the first place. If you have eaten a healthy meal where you got all your micro-nutrients: Carbs, Fats, and Proteins, you likely won't be hungry for a snack between meals. If you are eating clean, you most likely are no longer addicted to synthetic ingredients and MSG, and if you have broken your addiction to sugar (refer to my chapter on sugar in It Feels Good to Feel Good, Learn to Eliminate Toxins, Reduce Inflammation and Feel Great Again), then you won't be looking for snacks like you once were. These addictions turn off your hormones that regulate your appetite. But let's say you do want a snack, as a bridge between meals.

You will save a lot of money by making your snacks, and not buying either junk snacks or organic junk food. They add up to a lot of money with little nutrient benefit. Think in terms of making spiced nuts, or celery and nut butter, or already prepared cut up veggies on the top shelf of your refrigerator with homemade hummus (which takes minutes to make).[30,31] You can bake occasional treats like Danielle Walkers Real Deal Chocolate Chip cookies,[32,33] or NomNom Paleo's Cherry Chocolate Scones.[34]

You can also make your crackers, which are healthier than store-bought and don't take a lot of effort. By making your own, you also control that the ingredients are real food. Check my blog out on my website cherylmhealthmuse.com on foods for entertaining.[35]

5   Stop drinking soda and fruit juices.

If you want to stay away from pain, stop inflammation, and return to wellness, **NEVER** drink soda again. Drink water. Your body really, really needs water. You should add lemon or a few small pieces of fresh berries or fruit to your water and enjoy it that way instead. This also protects your electrolytes, according to my urologist. One-drop of Stevia makes it sweet. (I now use the powdered stevia leaf (ends up the alcohol in the stevia from the dropper wasn't so hot for me either.)[36]) Your body will thank you. And it's another important step to being well. If you do use liquid stevia, make sure it is just stevia. Many have dextrose in them, and dextrose IS sugar.

I ended up buying half-gallon glass bottles on Amazon,[37] and I make my own drinks. These drinks are infinitely more interesting. These are some of the things that I add to my glass bottle, with filtered water or sparkling water and keep cold in my fridge.

- Berries and peaches
- Blueberries, lemon, and cucumber
- Raspberries and mint
- Strawberries, kiwi, and basil
- Raspberries and lemon
- Watermelon, cantaloupe, honeydew
- Strawberries, mint, and orange
- Pineapple and ginger
- Cucumber and lavender
- Mint, basil, lavender, rosemary, and thyme
- Apple and cinnamon
- Tangerine, grapefruit, and strawberries

Using these tips saves money for real food and incorporates more real live food into your diet.

Now that you have found the money to spend on quality food, then let's talk about why this is so important.

This explanation was taken from a Cynthia Sass blog called, **"Why You Really Are What You Eat."**[38]

"The phrase, 'you are what you eat' is true. Nutrients from the foods you eat food provide the foundation of the structure, function, and integrity of every little cell in your body, from your skin and hair to your muscles, bones, digestive and immune systems. You may not feel it, but you're constantly repairing, healing, and rebuilding your body. Here's how it works, and why what you put on your plate is so important." Therefore, cooking your own food is important. By cooking, you control what you are feeding your body.

Your body is constantly repairing and producing new cells. Each part of your body has a different "shelf life." Your body produces these new cells based on the nutrients that you have been feeding it. You need a nutrient-rich environment to create healthy, vibrant new cells.

If you are eating "real" live food, then your body has healthy materials to utilize to replenish itself with strong and robust cells. If you are eating chemicals and synthetic ingredients from processed and fast food, or GMO's, then you are providing your body with poor construction materials to create the new cells, and eventually, this will impact the health of your body. You want your body to produce cells that operate optimally and that are less susceptible to aging and disease.

Your body is also replacing cells from the wear and tear of exercise and everyday life like stress, exercise, toxins, minor wounds, etc.

Under the best of conditions, this is the shelf life of each type of cell in your body:

- Your gut—the cells on your stomach and intestine wall live a hard life. They are constantly attacked by corrosives (stomach acid), as well as by toxins, parasites, candida, stress, mold, toxic metals, and pesticides and herbicides. These cells typically need to be replaced every six days. If these cells are constantly under attack, they begin to have a hard time keeping up. The gut is at the root of chronic illness, so it's important to keep producing healthy cells to rebuild your gut wall. Your gut wall is your line of defense to what is going through to your blood system.

- Your skin—the cells in your skin form the largest organ in your body. They live about 2-3 weeks.
- Your hair—the cells in your hair live about six years for women and three years for men.
- Your red blood cells live 3-4 months. This is the reason that when your doctor orders a sugar glucose test for diabetes, he gets an accurate reading. Some cells are new, some are in the middle of their life span, and some are getting ready to be replaced.
- Your liver—this critical organ is the detoxifier of your body. Contaminants go to your liver to be purified or removed. Your liver renews itself every 150-500 days. Be respectful of how much alcohol you drink, what pills you take, and how much sugar you eat. These things all impact the health of your liver, and it's critical to your long-term health.
- Your bones—although the cells in your bones are constantly regenerating, the complete process takes about ten years. The process to renew slows as we age, which is why bones begin to get thinner as we grow older.
- The brain—until recently, the scientific community believed that cells in the brain did not renew. It was discovered recently that the formation of new brain cells is not only possible but happens every single day. Polyphenols and flavonoids improve your brain's ability to regenerate.

I recommend that you "eat the rainbow." Whenever possible, eat your fruits and veggies organic. Avoid GMOs; you don't need the toxins that are used in their production. Each color of live food has a gift for your body, and miraculously, the colors all have different phytochemicals that work together synergistically to create a healthy body.

Eat the rainbow, without pesticides or herbicides, from a farm as close to you as possible (so that the nutrients are optimal). Eat in-season when these building blocks are their least expensive and in their prime health. Cook. This way, you control what goes into your body and the bodies of your children. As a result, your body can build healthy replacement cells. This is the key for your body to thrive. Give your body quality ingredients, and your body has all the right stuff to build healthy cells. Give your body garbage, and it's not a miracle worker, it can only do so much with what you are giving it.

This explains how a change to a healthier diet, and to cooking and eating real food improves how healthy your skin is, your energy level, and how you feel when you nod in with your body. I use the phrase; eating right makes your body sing. You need to nod in with your body and pay attention to how good real live food will make you feel. That's the power of eating for nutrients, and when you think about it, it's a downright miracle.

Buy organic. If your budget doesn't allow you to buy all your fruits and veggies organic, then follow the Dirty Dozen/ Clean 15 list that comes out every year.

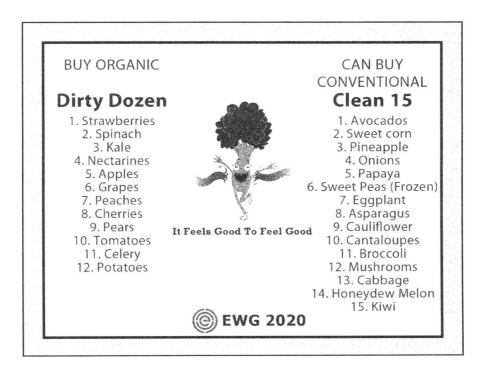

This list is published yearly by EWG at EWG.org. EWG stands for the Environmental Working Group. Get familiar with their site; it has a ton of fantastic information for your health.

If It is on the dirty side of this card, ONLY buy it organic. Otherwise, the fruit or veggie is loaded with tons of toxins. If it is on the Clean 15 side, you can buy it conventionally grown. EWG tests the toxins on these plants after scrubbing them many times. You cannot wash them off. You need to avoid all of them by choosing organic.

There is one other list to pay attention to, and those are what produce is now GMO. In my opinion, you do not want to eat GMO veggies and fruits. These either have BT Toxin bred right into the plant which is wreaking havoc on our body or these items have been grown "Roundup Ready" which means they have been engineered to be heavily sprayed with Glyphosate and it grows up into the plant, can't be washed off and has now been proven to cause cancer. Add these fruits and veggies to the items that you purchase organic.

For a complete explanation of GMOs, go to that chapter in my first book, It Feels Good to Feel Good, Learn to Eliminate Toxins, Reduce Inflammation and Feel Great Again.

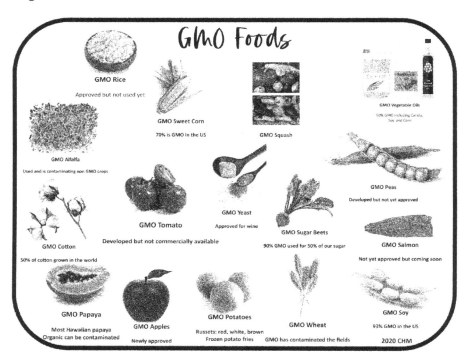

Chapter 6

Get to Know Your Farmer's Markets

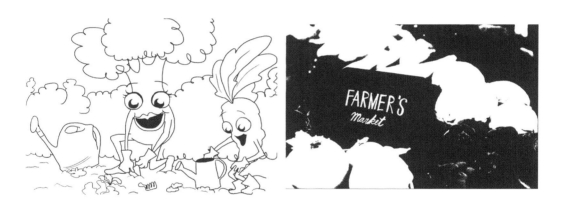

THE BIG TAKEAWAYS ON GETTING TO KNOW YOUR FARMERS MARKETS:[39]

- *By shopping farmer's markets, we find all kinds of healthy treats that wouldn't be available any other way.*

- *One of the best ways to find all the colors of the rainbow in season is to shop your farmer's markets. And yes, I do refer to them in the plural. There might be more than one in your area, and I think you should familiarize yourself with all of them. They all have different offerings.*

- *Visit all the farmer's markets in your area. There are different farmers and vendors at different markets, and you might find something wonderful that you would have missed had you only visited one.*

- *This is the easiest way to support your lifestyle commitment to eat all the colors of the rainbow, to get variety, to eat as close to the farm as possible, and to eat organic. Important even if you do not live on a farm.*

You now know that I believe you need to eat all the colors of the rainbow, from a farm as close to you as possible and that you should eat in season. I have even shared that three-quarters of your plate should be fruits and veggies at all meals. If it is on the dirty side of the dirty dozen list, you should eat it organic.

One of the best ways to do this is to shop your farmer's markets.[40] And yes, I do refer to them in the plural. There might be more than one in your area, and I think you should familiarize yourself with all of them.

John and I love to shop at farmer's markets. It's a fun thing that, whenever possible, we do together. We eat super healthy, and we are foodies, so by shopping farmer's markets, we find all kinds of healthy treats that wouldn't be available any other way.

One of the questions that I get asked is, "how do you make what you eat interesting?" To begin, it starts with having wonderful ingredients on hand when you go to your kitchen to cook. One of the things we do is shop for food at farmer's markets. We get outside and enjoy walking around in nature; we find places to explore for foods that are difficult to find or that we haven't eaten before. We get to know our farmers and ask them directly how they grow our food, preferably without pesticides and herbicides. And we find unique foods that are healthy, and that keeps life interesting.

One of our favorites is organic zucchini blossoms. They are available for a short-selling season, and they are a joy to add to our menu, whether it's just for us, or whether we have company over to enjoy them with us.

I like to stuff them with almond ricotta cheese (Kite Hill) that I add Italian herbs and a touch of marinara, and I add some vegan cheese that tastes like parmesan by VioLife. I then dip them in beaten egg (pastured free run eggs) and dip them in an organic all-purpose flour. (I don't want the Glyphosate that is on our conventional wheat.) I season the flour with a lemon and herb sea salt that I buy from a different farmer's market in the area. I then use organic onion and garlic powder and a touch of steak seasoning mix by Primal Palate. The steak seasoning is my secret culinary weapon. I pan fry them in ghee, put them in a pan and into the oven to keep them warm and crispy until they are all ready to eat. I then drizzle a little marinara sauce over them. They are amazing. I have never seen zucchini flowers in a regular market. They are fragile and have a short shelf life. But they are a true culinary delight. I do find them occasionally on the menu in high-end gourmet restaurants but usually made with ingredients that I don't eat.

I love my sea salt, and I love that it includes different herbs, so I use less salt when I am cooking. I buy it in Laguna Beach at their farmer's market.

At our Camp Verde farmer's market in Sedona, we can buy incredible organic loaves of bread that are amazing. I used to think I was gluten sensitive. Ends up, I am Glyphosate sensitive (the Roundup that our conventional wheat is drenched in for increased yield) And, there is a retired couple that grows their veggies. They will make me homemade V-8 that is delicious sans any chemicals.

Camp Verde also has beef from a rancher that is half the price of Whole Foods, and completely grass-fed, grass finished. He, too, has an autoimmune disease, so he is very picky about what he feeds his cows. And his beef taste is superior to any other beef I have ever eaten.

At our Sedona Up Town farmer's market, we can get direct from a shepherd lamb that melts in your mouth and has a very mild flavor when I cook it. This market also has a vendor with canned strawberries or blueberries, and I keep them in my pantry for when berries are no longer in season. I use them for syrup without the sugar.

We get all kinds of different apples at different farmer's markets. We get almonds that haven't been "pasteurized" with propylene oxide, directly from the ranch. US law insists all brands of almonds be "pasteurized." Most almonds are pasteurized with propylene oxide, or PPO which is related to formaldehyde, which in not good for us. A few almonds are pasteurized using steam. Only local growers are exempt from the law.

We get organic onions and garlic at most of our frequented farmer's markets. Buying our garlic from our farmers market is important because if you read about how garlic, in particular, is grown overseas, it's pretty disgusting. By buying organic at my farmer's market, we get goodness instead of who knows what on the veggie.

You can find different varieties of fruits and veggies at a farmer's market. These would be impossible to find at your local grocery store.

We can buy local honey at all these farmer's markets. This is important to reduce hay fever. Both John and I have struggled with hay fever, and by eating local honey, whether we are in California or Sedona, local honey has allowed our bodies to boost our immune system. (And as I have discussed elsewhere, we both take quercetin which has significantly reduced all our allergic reactions.)

I have learned about different types of olives that go into local California olive oil, and I prefer their taste. (And California law controls that olive oil is pure olive oil, so the mafia hasn't had a chance to dilute our olive oils with inferior vegetable oils.)

I have a fantastic fishmonger at my main farmer's market in Pasadena, and her fish is the freshest I have ever bought (and I lived in Seattle at one point). Fresh fish is much milder in flavor and worth the cost, especially if it is wild.

There are all types of eggs available. Ask the farmer how he treats his chickens. You want them outside as much as possible, and you want them eating their natural diet of grasses and bugs for the best-tasting eggs that are super healthy. Chicken, duck, and goose eggs are often available.

Fun and interesting varieties of mushrooms are available at all our farmer's markets.

You can buy plants at some farmer's markets for your garden.

You can buy organic mulch and fertilizer as some farmer's markets. And our farmer's market in Pasadena, CA, sells worms for gardening.

And of course, lots of luscious fruits and vegetables that are in season are in abundance from a variety of different farms.

Although you may be in a different part of the country from me, I would bet that there are wondrous finds at your farmer's markets as well. Make it an adventure and visit all the markets you can find in your area. In my opinion, farmer's markets make eating healthy fun and add variety to our diets.

Be prepared to eat what you purchase quickly, or, opt to freeze what you purchase for future eating. Organic produce spoils more quickly. It hasn't had additives in the growing process that are not good for you, and the purpose of those unhealthy additives is to slow down the aging process. You don't want fruit or veggies that have these additives, so it is not a bad thing that your fresh produce does not have them, it is a good thing, but plan accordingly.

What are the other advantages of shopping at a Farmer's Market?

1   It's the closest you will get to "farm to table" unless you shop directly at the farm.

    Usually, what is at the farmer's market was harvested the day before, or sometimes even the morning of, so you are getting the maximum amount of nutrients that that plant has to share with you.

2   You can get to know your farmer.

Talk to them about their farming practices, their use of herbicides and pesticides, their commitment to growing toxin-free produce. Not all the farmers I buy from are Certified Organic, which is a very expensive bookkeeping proposition, but most of these farmers are committed to a healthy growing environment. And I am a city girl, so this is a wonderful way to get to know the farming practices of my food.

Ask if you can visit the farm and learn more about their growing practices.

3 Often the price is much lower than what you are buying at your area's grocer.

At the farmer's market, you are buying what is in season, so you are buying what is in abundance. The same rules of supply and demand apply here, what is in abundance is the least expensive to buy.

4 Go early

You will find the largest selection if you arrive right after the farmer's market opens, and you get to pick from the best they have to offer.

5 Go late

By going at the end of the market, there might be a price advantage. Since they put them on the truck to get them to the market and they don't want to take them home again, one of our markets discounts the veggies and fruits that are leftover at the end of the market. This is not always the practice, but it's worth finding out.

6 There is often a local rancher at the market as well.

We only eat pastured meats. We eat Grass-Fed, Grass-Finished beef, Heritage pork that is pastured, pastured free-run chicken, and pastured eggs. You become what your animal eats, and you don't need a healthy dose of hormones and antibiotics that factory-farmed animals are given. You also don't need the stress hormones that a factory farmed animal has in their system because of the nasty way that factory farming treats animals. You want to eat animals that eat their species-specific diet without chemicals and that are humanely treated.

7	There are often other lovely things sold at the Farmer's Market that you won't get anywhere else.

As noted above, at one farmer's market, we buy beautifully canned (mason jars) organic tomato products, including salsas, and a wonderful V-8 type juice without all the ingredients that I can't pronounce (which are not good for me.)

We buy canned jams and jellies often made with less sugar and organic fruit.

As noted above, we also find organic bread at two of our markets that are out of this world. We only eat organic bread to avoid the healthy dose of Glyphosate (Roundup) that is now proven to be toxic that is sprayed on conventional wheat.

And another farmer's market has a vendor that cans berries, so that in the winter, I have those to make syrups, etc. with rather than frozen fruit. Again, organic and in glass Mason jars.

8	Farmer's markets are a wonderful place to find like-minded people.

Since we do not eat the SAD in my family (the Standard American Diet), we sometimes feel like we are swimming upstream. Others in our lives do not understand our commitment to high-quality toxin-free food, or why we don't eat processed or fast foods or eat out in restaurants regularly. I discuss how we handle this in another chapter. However, we have made many friendships that have become lasting from conversations with like-minded people at the farmer's markets.

9	And the biggie, which I want to repeat, is to buy as close to the farm as possible, and to eat all the colors of the rainbow and in season.

When you shop at a farmer's market, express your gratitude. People who sell at these markets need to drive great distances to bring you their produce; they wake up very early to arrive and set up their booths. We are fortunate to be able to buy their bounty directly from the farm.

Each color has a gift for your body, and all the colors work together synergistically to bring you health. Real Live Food Heals. Eat Organic.

If you live in an area that doesn't have year-round farmer's markets, I will discuss your options in the next chapter about where to buy high-quality food.

Part III

Living in Community

Chapter 7

Eating Healthy Out in Restaurants

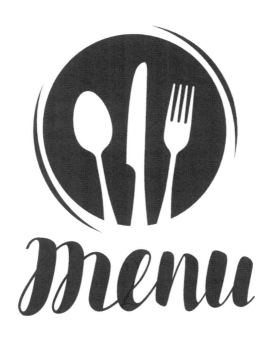

Menu

THE BIG TAKEAWAYS ON EATING OUT IN RESTAURANTS:[41]

- *Learning about what foods my body was sensitive to, and then avoiding them, was my first big step back to a world without pain.*

- *Whether or not you have sensitivities of your own that you avoid (see my chapter on sensitivities in my first book for a full explanation), or you have autoimmune disease, or you are a cancer survivor, or you have heart disease or even if you are healthy or a parent who wants to feed her children healthy food, understanding restaurants and how to eat out healthy is also important for you.*

- *I have 15 food sensitivities, so to start, I have printed a business card with all my sensitivities. (Vista Print. My picture is on it so that the waiter remembers who gave it to him.) These are foods that make me have a "flare," which in autoimmune terms means I react to them, and they make me gain a lot of weight overnight. They used to also bring me horrific pain.*

- *I check out menus online before we head out to any restaurant, and then I call them before we go to make sure I am safe.*

- *I do my research before I choose a restaurant; first, I get to know the owner over the phone, and then I am not afraid to ask for what I want.*

- *Keywords to look for when researching for a restaurant:*
  - *Organic*
  - *Farm to Table*
  - *Vegan, but sometimes those are problematic because Soy is a sensitivity. (and 95% GMO)*
  - *Happycow.net Happy Cow is a website that allows you to find vegan and vegetarian restaurants and health food stores across the world.*
  - *Grass-Fed/ Pastured*
  - *Wild fish*

- *See my additional tips to determine a restaurant so you can eat healthily.*

- *You don't want to be ravenous. You will make poor food choices, so eat something small ahead of going out.*

- *Don't be afraid to ask for exactly what you want. Be polite but be forceful.*

Learning how to eat out at restaurants has been an important skill for me to relearn. I will admit, I am hard to feed. I have 15 food sensitivities and won't eat ingredients that I know to be harmful to my body. Eating out is easiest when it is just John and me, and we get to control where we are going to eat. But we are both very social, so eating out with friends has also been an important skill to learn.

Learning about what foods my body is sensitive to, and then avoiding those foods, was my first big step back to a world without pain. So, I will always need to avoid these foods even when we eat out at all restaurants. I call my sensitivities my kryptonite, and I avoid them like the plague.

So why is this chapter important for everyone else to read?

Whether or not you have sensitivities of your own that you avoid (see my chapter on sensitivities in my first book for a full explanation)[42], or you have autoimmune disease, or you are a cancer survivor, or you have heart disease or even if you are healthy or a parent who wants to feed her children healthy food, understanding restaurants and how to eat out healthy is also important for you.

I have 15 food sensitivities, so to start, I have printed a business card with all my sensitivities. These are foods that make me have a "flare," which in autoimmune terms means I react to them, and they make me gain a lot of weight overnight (water weight-inflammation). Until recently, the flare also was accompanied by pain in my joints and muscles. The "flare" is inflammation. Now that I have cleaned up what I put into my body and healed my leaky gut, I no longer get the pain, but I still don't want the flare, so I am very careful what I eat no matter where I am. On the next page is what my card looks like.[43]

This is probably the single smartest thing that I have done since I got autoimmune disease. I have so many sensitivities, sometimes I don't even remember to tell someone what they are, so I keep these in my purse in a separate business card holder and then hand them out when I need to. (These cards save the waiter from running back and forth from the kitchen to me.)

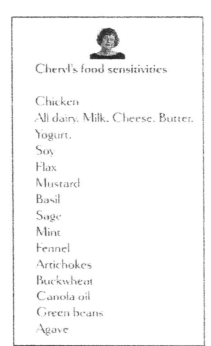

Cheryl's food sensitivities

Chicken
All dairy. Milk. Cheese. Butter.
Yogurt.
Soy
Flax
Mustard
Basil
Sage
Mint
Fennel
Artichokes
Buckwheat
Canola oil
Green beans
Agave

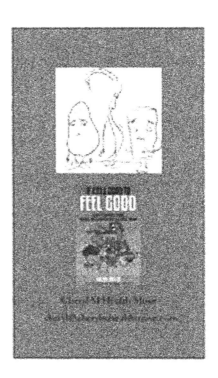

If you want to eat healthily, even if you don't have sensitivities, I recommend you print a card with things you truly want to avoid. It might be agave and canola oil for you, or things that are GMO, whatever it is, restaurants will react to a printed list and steer you away from unhealthy ingredients on your card.

When I hand these out in a restaurant or to a friend, I get a very positive reaction. Before I had the cards, I was sending the waiter back and forth to the kitchen as I remembered things, so this helps a lot.

As I have shared, I cook 90% of what John and I eat. That way, I KNOW what has gone into my food and its self-defense to make our food myself.

John has his own set of 13 sensitivities.

Despite all our restrictions, John and I are Foodies, and we love to eat good clean food.

I like to eat out as much as the next gal, so I want to share with you how we do that. This is especially tricky since neither of us eats the" SAD" any longer, which is the Standard American Diet.[44] (And it is a very sad diet and the way that most of America eats and the SAD is why I believe chronic illness is on the rise.)

To start, we live in Los Angeles, and we will travel for food. We go 40 miles north to Simi Valley to get a great fish dinner from our fishmonger (Marilyn's Mediterranean Kitchen) that sells us our fresh fish at our local farmer's market. We know she buys her vegetables organic from our farmer's market, and we trust that her "wild" fish is wild. Her family has been in the fish business for 30 years, and she knows her fish. If we do eat farmed fish from her, it is because we know it is sustainably farmed in the ocean without all the hormones and fake substances. We trust her.

Or, we might drive 1 hour across town to Venice to a vegan restaurant (Plant and Wine) that makes the most visibly beautiful meals I have ever seen.

There is a restaurant in Toluca Lake (Aeirloom Bakery) close to my Functional MD's office where I go for breakfast and lunch (closed for dinner). It is an organic bakery and does everything right. They use pastured eggs and bison and grass-fed, grass-finished beef and organic vegetables, and organic bakery goods. The baker will even bake me a pie at the holidays with ghee instead of butter and with maple syrup for the sugar and half the amount of sweet that the recipe calls for. These are standbys where I know I can get a delicious meal and not react. There is also a fantastic vegan restaurant in Studio City called Sun Café, which we enjoy, and it's the restaurant where we get takeout for guests at the Hollywood Bowl. (It is considered one of the top 10 restaurants in LA.) Many of their offerings are non-soy. All their food is clean and delicious.

Pasadena, close by, has a couple of restaurants I can enjoy carefully. I take my olive oil to have a salad at one because they use organic canola oil, which I do NOT want in my body.[45] They carry organic salads and grass-fed beef, so only the oil there is an issue. (Tender Greens)

There is also a vegan restaurant where there are a couple of dishes without Soy that I can eat. (Sage Plant-Based Bistro). Before I discovered that artichokes were a sensitivity for me, I used to order their artichoke appetizer and it is to die for.

I check all this out online before we head out to any restaurant, and I call them to make sure I am safe. We are also lucky to have a True Foods restaurant, which is Dr. Andrew Weil's restaurant, and there are offerings there that I can enjoy. His restaurant is beautiful, and his food is always delicious and clean.

We were given a gift certificate for a beautiful restaurant in South Pasadena, and I called the chef/owner ahead of time; he made sure that he could feed me organic and pastured meats, and he was thrilled to do it. We had a lovely meal there. I just had to give him a 24-hour warning that we were coming.

In Sedona, AZ, there are twelve restaurants that I can walk into right off the street, where the produce is organic, and farm to table and the meats are pastured. This doesn't mean that I can eat everything on their menus, but I can eat something very enjoyable at these establishments, and it is a pleasure to go out to eat there. My choices in Sedona range from organic vegan pizza[46], to healthy Mexican[47], to a new burger joint[48] close to where we live with organic buns and pastured beef. There is a restaurateur in the town named Lisa Dahl, and she has five restaurants[49] now where I can find something to eat that is clean. Her restaurants are also quite lovely, so she makes eating out something special. There is also a vegan restaurant[50] in town with all organic offerings and a beautiful garden in the back for dining. Feeding me in Sedona is easy, which is one of the reasons I am so happy we bought our second home there.

Mago, which is the Dao retreat outside of Sedona, is all organic and pescatarian, fish.

For very special occasions in Sedona, we go to the Enchantment Resort.[51] We are surrounded by red rocks there, that I feel I could almost touch from my table, and the food is farm to table and pastured. I had a beautiful meal there. We have not tried L'Auberge de Sedona yet, and although I could not order directly off their menu, I am sure that if I called ahead since they are farm to table, they could accommodate me.

The thing all the food above has in common is that I do my research; first, I get to know the owner over the phone, and I am not afraid to ask for what I want.

Now the question becomes, what do we do to scout out someplace new, or that is in a location where we haven't been before? These are the tips that I think will be most useful to you.

It starts with research.

Before I choose a restaurant, I research to see where I think I might be able to eat out. I am not shy about what I need and let everyone know this is for my health.

So, where to begin? The first thing that I Google are organic restaurants. Depending upon what comes up, I then check them out one by one. Often, they are NOT organic, or there is nothing to eat at that restaurant, so next, I google Healthy Food. Each step of the way, I look at the menus and see if there are things that I can eat at that restaurant. As I go, I make a list of possibilities.

Keywords I am looking for:

> Organic
>
> Farm to Table
>
> Vegan, but sometimes those are problematic because Soy is a sensitivity. (and 95% GMO) and many vegan restaurants are also heavily soy.
>
> **Happycow.net** Happy Cow is a website that allows you to find vegan and vegetarian restaurants and health food stores across the world.
>
> Grass-Fed/ Pastured
>
> Wild fish

I realize just because restaurants pop up in any of these categories; my research is not finished. Organic and Farm to Table are my best bet, but now I look at menus.

Tips when you are researching restaurants:

- Ask to speak with the chef, the owner, or the manager. Ask where the restaurant buys its produce.
- Ask what is made ahead and what is made to order. You can get a chef to change made to order items.
- Ask if they have any organic or grass-fed meat options.
- What are their healthiest dishes? It may or may not be something that you want to eat, but it's a great place to start.
- Ask what whole foods are available. This way, you know what you can order where they haven't added any unhealthy ingredients.
- Ask for steamed, poached, or roasted preparation
- Ask for wild-caught, pastured, organic, sustainable, locally sourced, or farm to table
- Don't be shy about asking if you can order "off" the menu. Let them know you will be requesting something simple and easy to make but clean. Explain that you eat very healthy. I share that I have autoimmune disease and sensitivities.
- I am not gluten sensitive. If you are, then you need to be asking about that too. I know that gluten sometimes is greater than just wheat, so learn about the cross sensitivities and add them to your list to inquire about.

Organic

If I can get an organic salad at the restaurant, I then call and ask about oils. Many restaurants use a canola/olive oil blend. 80% of canola oil is GMO. However, even if the canola oil is organic, it is not good for your health.[52] I read that the Canadians named it Canola because it comes from Canada and rhymes with Granola to make people think it is healthy. Read the note below. I call the restaurant and ask what they use. If it is a blend, then I take my olive oil in a small container or bottle. If I am in a restaurant and have not asked ahead of time, I ask to see the bottle. Remember, real olive oil has a greenish tint. The blends do not. In the worst-case scenario, I ask for lemon wedges and eat my salad with fresh lemon.

Farm to Table

These restaurants are usually a safe bet that there will be things I can eat. I still peruse the menu and, if necessary, call ahead and ask to speak to the owner or the chef.

Once we have chosen a restaurant, when we arrive, I give my sensitivity card to the waiter. I put my photo on it so that when he returns from the kitchen, he remembers who I am. The waiter will come and comment on what they have that might be ok, and since restaurants don't want a problem with allergies, they are especially careful.

Just a note: sometimes, they are overly cautious. John and I went to a Nobu in San Diego because I can always eat sashimi. I knew Nobu when we were both young, and he was starting out. I have enjoyed watching his amazing success. Well, they sent the chef to me to make sure that I wouldn't die if I came in contact with Soy. I assured them it was a sensitivity, not an allergy. (An allergy can kill. Where a sensitivity is a slow burn.) Then they sent the assistant manager over to talk to me—the same conversation. Finally, the manager approached me to tell me they couldn't feed me. Good grief, I pointed out they are a fish restaurant; of course, they could feed me. He still hesitated, so I pulled my "I know Nobu card." In the end, I had a marvelous dish that was soy-free and just wonderful. You must be pushy about what you want in both directions.

Sushi

Sushi is always a possibility, but I carry my non-soy soy sauce by Oceans Halo. It's not as good as soy sauce, but it doesn't have soy in it, which I react hostility to, so it works for me. It's also not GMO. When I eat out for sushi, I try for brown rice in my rolls, and then the fish. I don't eat things with cream cheese. I avoid the mayo, again usually made with Soy. I don't eat edamame. (GMO) or the miso (GMO). I avoid California roll unless it is made with real crab. The fake crab is not healthy for you. Sushi and sashimi are good choices.

"Do not order the seaweed salad, unless you know it does not contain food coloring. Food coloring is added to make that bright green color, as are additional harmful preservatives. Yellow #5 has the strongest link to severe allergic reactions, and Blue #1 has caused brain cancer in lab animals."[53]

How to Eat Healthy at Chinese Restaurants

- Ask for brown rice
- Ask for beef and broccoli with steamed veggies. Carrots are good, snow peas are good, without the sauce
- If you can eat chicken, then that is a good choice with the veggies too.
- Buddha's Feast with brown rice
- Ask what they can make for you without soy sauce.
- Ask if they use MSG in their food, and if they do, ask if they can make something without MSG.
- Carry your Dirty Dozen list with you at all times and avoid veggies on the list in your restaurant food.

We have a Chinese restaurant close that has soup dumplings. I eat those, and they are yummy. They also have many veggies which we order and are yummy. My most favorite thing is steamed dumplings. If they can make them without Soy, I go for it. I eat them with white rice wine vinegar. They are a treat. This restaurant does not use msg in their cooking. Ask.

Mediterranean

Mediterranean restaurants are usually a good bet because they have lamb and sheep eat grass. They also have hummus, which I can eat, and they have an eggplant dip that I can usually eat. Still important to ask what ingredients go into it. We recently went to one Mediterranean restaurant, and the eggplant dip had feta in it. Different countries call the eggplant dip different things. Sometimes it is called moutabel; sometimes, it is called Babaganoosh. SHIRAZI salad and tabbouleh are also good choices.

Greek salad full of fresh spinach, grilled chicken, or calamari with lots of fresh lemon juice and extra virgin olive oil drizzled on top. (I don't eat the chicken since I am sensitive to it, but you can. Chicken is an unusual sensitivity. I substitute calamari or shrimp if available.) If I'm really hungry, I order more grilled vegetables on the side. Since I am sensitive to dairy, I have them remove any feta. If I am going from home, I take a small glass container with my vegan feta crumbles in it to add to the restaurant dishes.

I recently had quail in a Mediterranean restaurant. They also offered frog legs. Both were done in olive oil, so they were both good choices. I wasn't crazy about the taste, but they were both "clean."

They also had grilled cauliflower on the menu, which reviews say is wonderful. That is something to try on another visit. Their rice was made with vegetable broth and was amazing.

Perk up grilled calamari, salmon, shrimp, or even a grilled whole fish with freshly squeezed lemon juice. Common fishes available in Mediterranean restaurants are Atlantic Salmon and Cod. Both are farmed and raised disgustingly, so I do not eat either.

"Souvlaki, plural souvlakia, is a popular Greek fast food consisting of small pieces of meat and sometimes vegetables grilled on a skewer. It is usually eaten straight off the skewer while still hot."[54] Souvlaki is another good choice.

Leg of lamb or lamb chops are a good choice.
Stay away from sauces.
You can usually find chicken, lamb, fresh fish, and shrimp dishes at a Mediterranean restaurant.

Mexican

A little harder to find healthy selections. There is a Mexican restaurant in Sedona that uses grass-fed beef, so I enjoy their Mexican food a lot. This Mexican restaurant is the exception to the rule. In other Mexican restaurants, a Fajita would be one of the better choices. Skip the sour cream and eat the guacamole instead. Ask for extra roasted veggies. I would skip the meat unless it is pastured. This is a time that I would eat beans for my protein. If you are dairy sensitive, you want to avoid the cheese. Ceviche is also a possibility in a Mexican restaurant.

Italian

A nice green salad with lots of roasted veggies would be a great start.

Pasta Fagioli is a good choice. I would need to ask if the soup base was chicken, at which point I would avoid it.

Fresh fish or seafood cooked in olive oil is a lovely entrée. You would want it to be wild fish or not fish that is farmed in chemicals.

Ask if the pasta is organic. Italian pasta does not have glyphosate in it.

Pasta Primavera good choice.

Pasta with marinara sauce is good. But the tomatoes are probably GMO. No cheese for me. If the cheese is imported, it will be without hormones, so go for it.

Di Mare—Shelled clams, black tiger shrimp, fresh garlic, Roma tomatoes, angel hair pasta, served in an olive oil white wine sauce. This is a possibility to ask the waiter about.

Ask for plain Italian pasta drizzled with olive oil, salt, pepper, and topped with steamed veggies.

Ask for a cheese-free pizza loaded with vegetables

I have found a wonderful vegan cheese with a strong parmesan flavor by VioLife. I have taken it with me to eat out. I shred it ahead of time and take it in a small jar.

Seafood

Unless it is a fine restaurant, most seafood has now been corrupted with chemicals. I do not eat Atlantic or Scottish salmon, which is farmed. The shrimp would be a better choice. They could also be farmed. Ask where they are sourced. You want them sourced in the Gulf of Mexico. I love Petrale Sole. Any wild fish is fabulous, like wild salmon or wild halibut. We love boiled crab type restaurants where they put the crab pieces right on the butcher paper in front of me. Eat vegetables like broccoli, cauliflower, and carrots that are not on the dirty dozen list.

> Note—If I am with a group of people, it helps if I have done my research ahead of time, and I then lead the group to a restaurant that I can eat at that they will enjoy too.

How to order food at a restaurant in general:

Once you are at the restaurant, you want to make sure you get a healthy meal.

Make sure you are not overly hungry. In my travel chapter (Chapter 12), I have listed travel food to have available to stave off that uncontrollable hunger feeling. Have a snack before you go out to dinner that is healthy, like an organic apple, and take the edge off before you even walk in the door.

You don't want to be ravenous. You will make poor food choices, so eat something small ahead of going out.

Don't be afraid to ask for exactly what you want. This is especially important if you haven't had a chance to call ahead.

Ask all the questions that you need to have answered about sourcing and preparation. I have found that restaurants will go out of their way to make me happy. Is it uncomfortable? A little at first, but it's your responsibility to know what you're putting into your body and your waiter's responsibility to know what goes into the food they're serving. The more you ask, the easier it gets, I promise!

I start by handing the waiter my card. I send him to the kitchen and ask him for the chef's recommendations.

Focus on eating REAL FOOD. Many restaurants now buy their food in baggies, and they warm up the food and arrange it on your plate. That food tends to be saucy and loaded with chemicals. Keep it simple. I have even carried ghee in a small jar in my handbag to whip out and use on steamed veggies. Ghee is butter that has had the milk solids removed, so there is no whey or casein in it, which is what I am sensitive to in dairy. Without the milk solids, it is very stable and doesn't spoil, so it travels well. And ghee is a healthy oil for autoimmune diseases.

Always ask if the soup is made from scratch. Avoid soups that use a pre-made base or even worse are straight out of a can. Pre-made bases can be full of MSG, loaded with salt and other artificial ingredients. In my case, I also ask if the base is chicken broth. Zoot, I can't go near chicken, since it has become a sensitivity.

Set your mind to stick to the principle learned from Blue Zones that you only want to eat until you are 80% full. You will be much better off, and your body will be happy. The easiest way to do that is to eat until you are just at the line of no longer being hungry. If you eat until your brain recognizes you are full, you probably have overeaten.

Instead of bread, ask the waiter for raw cut up veggies to start the meal. You don't need a dip, but it helps to have something crunchy to munch on.

Ask for water right away and get lemon to put into your water. Not all restaurants will automatically bring you water now unless you ask.

Once you know what the restaurant chef recommends for you to eat, ask for simple food preparation. Grilled or steamed preparation is great. Poached is also a good choice for fish whenever possible or grilled. Steamed, baked, roasted, braised, broiled, and seared are all good preparation methods.

Avoid any menu description that uses the words creamy, breaded, crisp, sauced, or stuffed as they are likely loaded with saturated fats. Other "beware of" words include buttery, sautéed, pan-fried, au gratin, Thermidor, Newburg, Parmesan, cheese sauce, scalloped, and au lait, à la mode, or *au Fromage* (with milk, ice cream, or cheese). Also beware of pan-fried, crispy, dipped, scalloped, breaded, creamed, and alfredo as they are not healthy cooking methods for you to eat.

Ask for olive oil to use on your food, but again ask to see the bottle to make sure it is truly olive oil. Nine times out of 10, it is a canola/olive combo 90/10, so make sure you know what you are using. Again, real olive oil is a green-tinged oil. I often carry my own in a small bottle, double bagged.

Instead of starches, ask for double veggies. I hesitate to eat even a baked potato out because of the 39 pesticides used on a conventional potato. I try to avoid the veggies on the Dirty Dozen (Strawberries, Spinach, Kale, Nectarines, Apples, Grapes, Peaches, Pears, Tomatoes, Celery, Potatoes, All Peppers, Cherry Tomatoes, Lettuce, Cucumbers, Blueberries, Plums) or the GMO list (Corn, Soy, Sugar (refined sugar (beets)), Papayas (from Hawaii), Canola).

Avoid sauces, dressings, and dips. These are usually laden with hidden sugars, unhealthy oils, gluten, and dairy.

Stick to reasonable portion sizes. If your plate has too much food on it, get a takeout box right away and put the extra food aside where you won't fiddle with it and end up eating it. (My father was one of those people who always told us people in Europe were starving, so I had to eat what was put on my plate as a child. It took me years to figure out that wherever the starving people were, they were starving whether I overate or not. I still catch myself moving food around my plate until it is gone. Better for me to remove it from my plate upfront.)

Eat mindfully and eat slowly. I used to end my day at the office at full speed and then sit down to eat my evening meal at full speed as well. Relax, enjoy the company of who you are with and be mindful of each bite and how delicious the natural flavors are.

I just read that one of the benefits of saying grace is that we slow down and signal our body that it is safe to eat and for our bodies to put attention on digesting our food. It is a form of gratitude, and either praying or gratitude are lovely traditions to have before a meal.

The other suggestion is to eat something bitter before the meal, like parsley or cilantro. That wakes up our stomach enzymes so that we get the maximum benefits from what we are eating.

Focus on protein and vegetables, no matter where you are eating.

Ask for berries for dessert.

Drink water or iced tea (unsweetened) with lemon—no colas, or sugary drinks

Hot tea is a good choice but be aware that paper bags are best. (Or loose) Those cute little triangular bags are plastic and emit toxins.

Now, if you are thinking I don't want to be this pushy when I go out to eat, I want to tell you a story.

John and I traveled to Ohio to visit with his family. We still stayed in hotels, so that we could control some of our food and our time. (See my chapter on traveling healthy (Chapter 9).)

There was a very special hotel, and restaurant that John wanted to share with me called The Golden Lamb in Lebanon, Ohio. The hotel and restaurant are 200 years old, and 12 US Presidents have stayed there. John knew how much I loved old places with history, so this was a must.

Besides, I had a friend from my jewelry days who lived just a little bit north, so we invited him to join us for dinner. We were going to eat there, so I was nervous about what the restaurant might be able to feed me.

As soon as we arrived (the day before our dinner), I spoke to the front desk about my dilemma and asked if I could speak to the head chef. He arranged a meeting that day.

When we met, and I gave the card to the chef, I will admit I was awkward and nervous. My company was coming no matter what.

He read the card, looked and me and smiled, and said, "Oh goodie, I get to cook something new and fresh and interesting. I get so bored always cooking the same thing. Just leave it to me."

So, we met our guest, and John and Michael ordered, and then the chef bought out our dinners himself. My meal was sensational and gorgeous and clean. Michael commented he wished he had known; he would have ordered my meal as well. But we all had a sensational meal, and everyone was thrilled.

There was nothing to be hesitant or embarrassed about, after all. So, ask. The worst thing that can happen is that they say no. My book coach is always saying, "get your ask on."[55] Don't be afraid to ask for what you need. Let them surprise you.

Since I have learned that eating out with friends is about enjoying their company and not about what I am eating, had he said no way, I would have eaten something ahead of time, and then enjoyed a salad while my friend and hubby ate.

I have similar stories to tell when I get to the chapter about traveling in Europe. The point is, ask for what you want, and then adjust accordingly.

Finally, sometimes I don't control where the party eats. Since I eat "clean" the rest of the time, I make the best possible choice from the menu as I can. Remember, it's all about toxic load. Don't get twisty. One meal won't kill me, and it won't kill you. If you are eating with friends, it's always about community, so enjoy the people you are with and don't make them uncomfortable about their food choices. Don't lecture them or judge what they choose to eat. Just eat as clean as possible. Remember, you always have your emergency food pack if you are hungry when the meal is over.

Chapter 8

Eating at Friends and Family Homes, Going to Parties

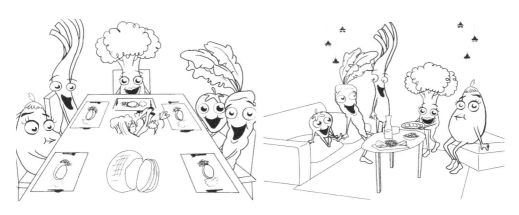

THE BIG TAKEAWAYS ON EATING OUT AT FRIENDS AND FAMILY HOMES:[56]

- *Community is an important part of health, so living in isolation is not the answer. Whether or not you have sensitivities of your own that you avoid (see my chapter on sensitivities in my first book for a full explanation), or you have autoimmune disease, or you are a cancer survivor, or you have heart disease or even if you are healthy or a parent who wants to feed her children healthy food, understanding how to eat out healthy is also important for you.*

- *I know it is not my role to judge or to lecture, and I do love being with all of the people I love, so depending upon how they eat makes a big difference in how we handle invitations.*

- *I will warn you, in the beginning, there was a fair amount of hostility from loved ones because they seemed to think that our eating "clean" meant that we were judging them. Being empathetic is an important part of loving relationships on both sides.*

- *I changed how I ate because of my health, and that silences the critics. For those of you that want to change before you get "sick and tired of being sick and tired," it takes conviction to jut up against how others eat.*

- *Community is about love, and food is not. This is a mindset shift that you must make.*

I dearly love my friends and family but must admit, most of them do not eat as we do. Community is an important part of health, so living in isolation is not the answer. We have no intention of living without our community, so we have had to find solutions for eating together.

Often, as a result, we will go out to dinner at a Cheryl approved restaurant instead of at someone's home. Food is thought of as love, and my friends and family often want to cook for us as well as their other friends, so finding ways to navigate around the food we will be served has been a journey.

Different friends and family fall into different categories in terms of how they eat. Understand, I know it is not my role to judge or to lecture, and I do love being with all of them, so depending upon how they eat makes a big difference in how we handle invitations. We always go, but we adjust according to how they are cooking.

I will warn you, in the beginning, there was a fair amount of hostility from loved ones because they seemed to think that our eating "clean" meant that we were judging them. Being empathetic is an important part of loving relationships on both sides. I do believe that how we eat would be good for all our loved ones, but also understand that it can take 17 touch points for someone to change. I know from my retail management days that if you push someone, they will push back. Not judging is a part of love. And that works in both directions.

I changed how I ate because of my health, and that silences the critics. For those of you that want to change before you get "sick and tired of being sick and tired," it takes conviction to jut up against how others eat. I do have a friend that has always eaten healthy, and when we changed how we eat, her response was, "thank goodness, now there are three of us." So, stand your ground, whatever your motivation, and stay the course.

I concluded right after I got sick and significantly changed how I eat, that community was about love and food was not. I could enjoy being with friends and family, whether they were eating and serving me food that I could eat or not. This is important because it is a mindset change that has made all the difference for me.

I try to accommodate loved ones when they come to our house for dinner without giving up on our eating standards. One family member doesn't like tomatoes, so I don't use them when I cook for her. Another loves pierogi, which I no longer eat, but if we are doing Polish food, I will have them available for her.

What they serve and eat at their home has nothing to do with me; what they eat doesn't mean that I must eat it. The joy and the love of being with them are what is important.

Therefore, for my family, I bought them all some of the Paleo cookbooks that I use when I cook. They know that if I am going to their home for dinner, this is a great place to start to cook for me. It's not a requirement, but they love me and don't want to feed me anything that might make me a "flare," so it's a loving thing for them to do to cook for me from these sources. This is my immediate family, so I did not feel "pushy" making this request.

However, not every invitation is from a friend or family member who will accommodate my eating habits, so now what do I do?

To start, I don't make a big deal about it, I find out what the hostess is serving, and then I make suggestions of dishes that I would like to bring to the dinner party. I make enough for everyone but know that this is probably what John and I will be eating that night at their house.

I make my crackers and dips, so I often offer to bring them. (I have a blog with the recipes I use on my website.)

People who know and love me realize this is about my health, so they understand that I want to bring food that I can eat.

Sometimes, John and I bring our version of what the party will be eating. As an example, if it's a birthday party for children, and they are eating hot dogs, then we bring Applegate hot dogs, cook them on the barbeque, and eat with everyone else. They are probably eating potato salad or pasta salads, so I make my pasta and potato salads, but a little different and most likely healthier, and everyone can also enjoy my version. My version is with Follow Your Heart Soy Free Mayo and organic potatoes, either red potatoes or russet, our plates look similar, and all is well. My pasta salads usually are loaded with organic veggies as well as organic pasta, and probably would have an oil (olive or avocado) and vinegar base. I make a great black bean salad loaded with chopped up veggies and olive oil and vinegar that is delicious. I make yummy food that is cleaned up from the SAD (standard American diet) version. And I avoid all GMO vegetable oils.

We once went to a pizza party, so we made our pizza, on a Capello's almond flour crust, with roasted veggies and Applegate pepperoni (for John) and Applegate ham (on the other half for me) and organic pineapple. We cooled and cut it ahead of time, and then slid it back into the original box. We topped it with organic arugula. When all the pizzas arrived, we put our slices on our plates and ate with everyone else.

I love to make salads of all the colors of the rainbow in a great big glass bowl that I own. This is a favorite at our family Christmas party. It's a ton of work and chopping, but we all get to enjoy the beauty of the colors and the goodness of all the nutrients, and it's become requested huge hit.

I went to a friend's home when I was starting to explore different ways to cook healthy, and I took a big bowl of zucchini noodles and raw tomato sauce. It was so popular with her guests that there was almost none left for me, so I have learned now to take my food in a separate container and to also take a big container of the dish for everyone else. I have discovered that if the food is delicious, then healthy is a plus, and people will be more than willing to try it, even if it strikes them as weird.

When we invite company to our home, I try to cook things that they may not have previously tried. One of my favorite things to make is cauliflower rice. I have now made it Moroccan (with cumin and cinnamon that gets toasted in ghee before I start the rest of the dish and fills the entire house with an incredible smell) and then add raisins, cherries, apricots, roasted slivered almonds, roasted garlic and onion. I also have made it Italian, with Italian seasoning (Primal Palate, called Amore), sundried tomatoes from Trader Joe's, Italian green olives, and yellow bell pepper. We have found a delicious parmesan vegan cheese that I add. I have made it Greek, with parsley, tomatoes, Greek olives, sundried tomatoes, and vegan feta cheese, etc. I even made paella with it once with saffron and all the appropriate seafood. I match the pastured meat or wild fish to the dish. There is always a big salad with homemade salad dressing, and often additional vegetables.

Again, I have discovered if the food is delicious, people love that it is also healthy. As a result, I am not afraid to feed them super healthy exactly like John, and I eat. Being a foodie, my cooking is delicious, if I do say so myself.

We have also had pizza parties, where I have all kinds of toppings, made ahead of time[57], and everyone gets their half or whole Capello's pizza crust to make their pizza. It's fun, and all the ingredients are healthy. We don't all eat at the same time because it takes time for each pizza to cook, but no one has complained because they are getting it "their way." We have great conversations waiting for each "pie" to be ready. (We have a steel pizza slab that gets the crust nice and crunchy.)

We have also done a great job of converting old family favorites to new healthy versions. At Christmas time, we have John's family over for Golabki, a Polish favorite, and we have cleaned up all the ingredients. We have someone in Sedona that makes and cans homemade V-8 juice for us, so that is the base, and we play Use This Not That with the rest of the recipe. I then make Polish vegetable salads, and it's a great meal to share in community with loved ones. This is where we also cook perogy for the rest of the family, even though we don't eat them. Maybe someday I will learn to make them from scratch with all organic ingredients.

I make a mean almond flour chocolate chip cookie (Danielle Walker Read Deal Chocolate Chip Cookies) that all my friends love, so I will often bring them to the occasion. I am often asked to bring my chocolate chip (no soy, Enjoy Life chocolate chips) dried cherry almond flour scones. (Recipe by Nom Nom Paleo)

I have an organic bakery, and I can get things there for dessert that we can eat, and that company loves. Most often, we serve berries for dessert with whipped coconut cream, so what's not to love about that?

One last thing, I am often asked to bring organic bread. I thought I was gluten sensitive, ends up I am glyphosate (Roundup) sensitive, so organic bread is a treat for all. Whole Foods has organic bread, and I have a bakery both in Pasadena with lovely organic loaves of bread and in the Sedona area where I can get amazing organic bread.

If we are going somewhere where we don't know the hostess well, and we are not sure of the food, we eat the salad and eat from our emergency pack. Again, it is for my health, so I explain that it has nothing to do with her cooking. I stay firm in what I will put into my body, and everyone seems to understand. If I need to, I explain my philosophy that community is about love and not about food, and that takes the edge off.

CATERING

Where there is a will, there is a way. We catered my book party for my first book, and we will cater again when I finish this book and reintroduce the new, updated, and edited first book. John has friends at a small local butcher and grocer, and they catered it using completely organic ingredients and healthy appetizers. It wowed our guests, and it was spectacular. We have already approached a local restaurant about holding our next book signing party at their establishment, and they are eager to give it a whirl. They have many organic offerings now, so it is a natural to throw our party there.

When John and I got married five years ago, we got married privately in a friend's backyard. We then threw a party at a sensational restaurant up in the Malibu mountains called Saddle Peak Lodge. We chose this restaurant because of their commitment to farm to table vegetables, and their wild meats on their menu that eat their species-specific diet. It was a luncheon and all organic. It was a reception to remember. They have a large open patio, surrounded by beautiful trees and nature and a space large enough that the kids could play freely at one end of the porch away from the adults, and yet they were completely protected. The food was spectacular. Once you commit to eating differently from the rest of America, it is do-able. The ad slogan that I eat "delicious, nutritious, and nothing suspicious"[58] has served us well when we are entertaining.

I enjoy the company no matter what I am eating; I remain firm about what I put into my body. Enjoying my community is the point of getting together.

Part IV

Travel

Chapter 9

Healthy Travel - Planes, Trains, and Automobiles

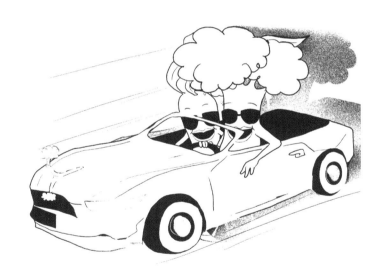

THE BIG TAKEAWAYS ON HEALTHY TRAVEL—PLANES, TRAINS, AND AUTOMOBILES:[59]

- *Travel takes planning. Yes, I know you plan for your flights and your rental car if you are flying, but you now also want to plan out how you will be healthy in your new location. I do this at least two weeks before I go anywhere.*

- *Whether or not you have sensitivities of your own that you avoid (see my chapter on sensitivities in my first book for a full explanation), or you have autoimmune disease, or you are a cancer survivor, or you have heart disease or even if you are healthy or a parent who wants to feed her children healthy food, understanding restaurants and how to eat out healthy is also important for you.*

- *Locate where the closest organic grocery stores are to buy healthy food before you book your hotel room.*

- *You will want to book your hotel, keeping in mind what you want to see while you are there, and where you can conveniently get the food that you will eat.*

- *Book a hotel room that comes with a refrigerator.*

- *Avoid airplane food.*

- *It's important to get up and move every hour or two on an airplane. Walk and bounce.*

- *Do not eat processed or fast food.*

- *Carry a snack emergency kit.*

Travel takes planning. Yes, I know you plan for your flights and your rental car if you are flying, but you now also want to plan out how you will be healthy in your new location. I do this at least two weeks before I go anywhere.

Booking a hotel room

1. Map out where you are going. If you are going to an event, find where it is on a map. If you are visiting friends or family, you still need to do the same thing. Get a feeling for the lay of the land.

    Next, before you book your flight or your hotel room, you will want to find healthy food.

2. Locate where the closest organic grocery stores are to buy healthy food. Most cities have Whole Foods, many have Sprouts, and if not, there is someplace in the town where there are organic produce and groceries. Know where these outlets are before you take your next step.

3. If there are no Whole Foods or Sprouts available, get as much information as you can for an alternative store. If they have a website, check it out. If you can't get enough information online, call the store and talk to the store manager to ensure that you can get the food that you need.

4. Now you will want to book your hotel, keeping in mind what you want to see while you are there, and where you can conveniently get the food that you will eat.

5. Book a hotel room that comes with a refrigerator. Check out Residence Inns first, because they also come with a kitchen. At a different brand hotel? Don't book the room until they confirm they have a small fridge that they can reserve for the room. When you check-in, ask if they have put it into the room. I call if possible before I leave for my flight to remind the hotel that I need the fridge. Ask them to clean the refrigerator out. You don't want their snacks, liquids, and alcohol. This will leave you room for your healthier food. (and you won't "bump" their food, making it register as eaten and purchased. You don't want their stuff charged to your room, so this avoids that 100%).

6. Now I book my flight and my car. Make sure that you will arrive with plenty of time to swing by the designated organic grocer to pick up healthy food for the visit.

The trip itself

7. Take some band-aids in your luggage if you are going to be walking more than normal. They can be a lifesaver.

8. Avoid airplane food. Don't eat the snacks handed out on the plane. They are empty calories and give no nutrition to your body. Airline nuts are in vegetable oils, so you don't want them. See below; you are going to have your snack pack, so what the airline offers to you is unnecessary.

9. I have a blow-up neck pillow that takes up little room but comes in handy to be comfortable in an airline seat.

10. Wear compression socks. I have a problem that my ankles swell when I am on airplanes, and compression socks keep my legs and ankles comfortable.

11. It's important to get up and move every hour or two on an airplane. If I walk back to the bathroom on a plane, inevitably someone is using it, so I use that time to bounce and get the blood flowing through my body.

12. When I used to travel often to Asia for my jewelry business, one of the things I loved about Northwest Airlines[60] was we all did airplane aerobics in Business Class before the plane landed. I wish I had filmed it. You do the exercises seated, and most of them are resistance exercises or tapping exercises. Stretch, do exercises like my 2-minute stress releasing exercises from your airline seat. (see my chapter on stress in this book, Chapter 12.) Tap as far down on your legs that you can reach and go all the way up to your head and then back down. Get the blood flowing through your limbs and back up to your brain. You shouldn't care if you look silly, it's good for you and if people are staring, smile and invite them to join you. Your body will thank you that you woke it back up before you gather your things after you land to get off the plane.

13. If your flight is going to arrive too late to shop, take a refrigerator bag with icepacks on to the plane. I own several that I use for shopping at farmer's markets on weekends, they are insulated, and with ice packs (re-freezable ice packs can be bought at a camping goods store), they keep the food cold. Check the food as baggage. Take Vital Farms, organic pastured hard-boiled eggs (Sprouts sells them cooked) or another brand of pastured eggs that you have hard-boiled, seasonal fruit, a salad from

your local Whole Foods Salad bar, Applegate ham and Applegate turkey cold cuts (your cold cuts should be closest to the ice packs). Take organic bread. Avoid regular bread because of the density of glyphosate (Roundup) on the wheat. Organic tortillas are a great substitute for organic bread and easy to use for sandwiches.

14. Take a Mason jar stuffed with a towel (to keep it from breaking) to make a salad for lunch. Take it on the plane with you in your carry-on luggage so that it doesn't break, but you have it on your trip.

15. Airlines allow a quart-sized bag of liquids, aerosols, gels, creams, and pastes in your carry-on bag and through the checkpoint. These are limited to travel-sized containers that are 3.4 ounces (100 milliliters) or less per item. Carry salad dressing of olive oil, seasonings, lemon juice, and Braggs apple cider vinegar in small bottles that can go through airport security. Or, place them in secure baggies and pack them in your insulated bag. I usually use more than one baggie so that I don't get the oil all over everything in my travel bag. Don't forget to squeeze all the air out of the baggies.

16. I like to carry bamboo utensils and plates with me when I am on the road.

17. Do not eat processed or fast food. (There are no nutrients in them. There are toxic ingredients in them.)

18. Carry a snack emergency kit. Do not get into a situation where you are starving and then make bad choices to get something to eat. I also always have an emergency kit in my car at all times when I am tootling around town. This is the same "emergency pack" that I carry onto planes or in the car when we travel. I never will eat fast food again, except for an occasional Chipotle, and I can stick to that conviction because I am always prepared.

Include protein bars (with no soy, no GMO's, low sugar, no corn syrup or fructose), and salmon jerky (no soy).

Enjoy Life has wonderful 70% (or 68% chocolate) snacks that are soy-free for a sweet treat.

Dried fruits from the Ugly Co. is a new product on the market that is making use of bruised and distorted apricots, peaches, and kiwi. The peaches are on the Dirty Dozen list so that I won't eat those, but the apricots and kiwi are a wonderful snack. Their goal is to lower food waste, and I applaud them. Their product is delicious. The hard end of the kiwi is on the end of the dried piece, so I bite it off before I eat it.

Carry organic nuts. (organic almonds, organic pecans, or walnuts. Sunflower seeds and pumpkin seeds)

Include a can or 2 of wild salmon in your pack. Careful when you open the can. (I once sprayed the oil from the can all over me and smelled like cat food until I got off the plane and could change).

Always have packets of Artisana nut butter in the emergency food supplies, a great source of protein, and yummy spread on fruit.

http://bit.ly/travelpacknutbutters

Include fruit that is in season and a banana in your emergency supplies. I always have a couple of green organic apples with me. I also carry celery, it's a great way to eat nut butter and adds a little crunch.

19. Research the restaurants in the area to see what options are available before the trip begins. Look at the online menus and call the restaurant owners about possible options for healthy eating. Look for words like "farm to table," "wild-caught fish," "pastured or grass-fed beef," "local lamb" (grass is their normal diet), "pastured or free-run chicken," "local, sustainable." Ask what oils they use and restrict your use to olive oil (and ask to see the bottle to make sure it is not an olive/ canola mix. If necessary, pack another small glass bottle with real olive oil. Pack a bottle of ghee.) Inquire if steamed veggies, poached fish, and poached eggs are an option.
20. If there are no good options, to join family or friends at dinner, eat from your emergency food, and still join the party. I have discovered that being with a loving community has nothing to do with the food that I choose to eat. Enjoy the company and the community without the food.

You can take your food into the restaurant and order your drink. I have never once had a restaurant complain.

21. You should pack stainless-steel bottles with filtered water in your luggage. Plastic leaches chemicals into the water, so carry your own stainless. The chemicals from plastic are harmful. If I am going to be gone for several days, when I am at the grocery store, I buy spring water in jugs. I know it is in plastic, but at least I am not drinking out of the hotel tap.

22. In the morning, in your room, make your organic coffee using a single serving French press gismo. Coffee is sprayed with tons of herbicides and pesticides, so this ensures a chemical-free cup freshly brewed. I carry my organic coffee with me. I prefer the taste of my brand anyway, so I take it along.

    http://bit.ly/singlecoffeepress

23. I have a morning exercise routine. It takes no equipment and can be easily done while I am on the road. It starts with me stretching before I even get out of bed. I stretch the full length of my body, and then twist my knees to one side with my head to the other and then I reverse it. When I pop out of bed, I also stretch, first reaching up to touch the ceiling and then dropping down to touch my toes, and I hold the stretch.

24. Most hotels have a gym, so plan time to go work out on the equipment before you start your day. It will get the blood flowing in your body.

25. If possible, I have bought a salad at the grocery store organic salad bar. I now get my Mason jar, and I make my lunch. I put my Applegate cold cuts and my sliced hard-boiled eggs on top. I pop one of my bottles of oil and vinegar into my bag and secure both in multiple plastic bags. I buy all sizes of baggies from Paper Mart, a carryover from my jewelry days. I carry big bags with me that can fit smaller baggies into them.

26. Don't eat at the breakfast buffet. The eggs are loaded with chemicals. If you do go downstairs to the buffet, stick to the fresh fruit that they have for you. Pick up a couple of pieces of fruit and eat your hard-boiled eggs.

27. If traveling by car, do all the above except take along a small refrigerator from Amazon to keep food cold on the way. It plugs into the car. This is not very large, but you can keep your chicken or cold cuts cold while

you are on the road. We picnic when we travel by car, so we find a great park if possible. If we are traveling between LA and Sedona, we have a favorite rest stop in the middle of the desert where we stop and picnic. If we are traveling where we need to buy food, we get it at a grocery that has organic food, and preferably an organic salad bar.

http://bit.ly/travellfridge

Other tips to stay healthy:

- Take your shampoo and conditioner in small travel sizes. Cosmetics and hair products are unregulated and loaded with toxins. Currently, I am using Pacifica vegan products and their travel sizes of Super Kale Juiced-up Shampoo and Super Kale Juiced-Up Conditioner (2 oz).

  http://bit.ly/pacificatravelsz

- Carry your mini squirt bottle of hand soap in the pocket of your pants. There are toxins in public bathroom hand soaps. I use a travel sized Soapwalla hand, and body wash. It comes in 3 flavors. Recover, Recharge, or Comfort. The bottles are small enough to be in my pant pocket so that I always have them. They are easy to use and squirt out the right amount of soap onto my hands. My hands break out from the chemical soaps in public restrooms, but even if you don't have this problem, avoid the toxins from going into your skin. AVOID ANTIBACTERIAL SOAPS, they are loaded with toxins, and they grow bacteria. Soap and water are your best bet to stay. Hot water is even better with soap.

  http://bit.ly/travelsoapwalla

- I also travel with Soapwalla travel-sized deodorants. Completely non-toxic, and they work. They are made with clay and essential oils. I use the regular size at home, and she now offers a flavor for sensitive skin. (She has MS or Lupus, so making products that she could use, became her mission).

  http://bit.ly/traveldeoderant

My last tips:

- Make sure you still get at least 7 hours of sleep. It is very important to your long-term health. I use the Dr. Andrew Weil 4-7-8 breathing exercise to relax my body, which helps me fall asleep. I seem to have trouble falling asleep when I travel east, and not when I travel west (there is a theory that when you travel against the sun, it fiddles with your circadian rhythm. I have tons of ghee jars stored in my home, so I fill one up with Epsom salts to use in the hotel bathtub, and I take a bath to help me relax. I also carry a lavender essential oil to add to the bath for additional relaxation.
- In any kind of a stressful situation, use the Dr. Andrew Weil 4-7-8 breathing exercise to calm yourself and reset your parasympathetic nervous system. You can watch a YouTube video of Dr. Weil on your phone and do the exercise with him. The entire exercise takes 3 minutes, and it releases stress before it begins to accumulate to a chronic state.

  http://bit.ly/weilbreathing

- If you are going to be outside, don't forget to apply sunscreen. Sunscreens can be very toxic, so make sure that what you use has clean ingredients. I use a face cream from KeysPure that is an SPF 30+ to protect my face, and I use Pacifica Beauty sun care. It comes in a mini size, so it doesn't take up too much space to travel. More on sun care in another chapter (Chapter 15).

  http://bit.ly/lowtoxinsunscreen

- I always carry lavender/tea tree oil in my cosmetic bag. I use it, if I need it, to repel insects. It has worked for me in Asia dealing with unknown bugs, and domestically for mosquitos. I will admit it doesn't smell the best, but better than having hundreds of bites, which happened to my business partner once. At the first bite, I put tea tree all over my exposed skin. My partner said yuck and refused. By the time we got to our next stop, I only had the one bite, and she was covered from head to toe. I also carry KeysPure Insect repellant on me and keep it at home. It is an amazing product. When I get the first bite, this product soothes the bite, and then I use it on all exposed skin, and for me, it works. The tea tree oil is easier to carry in my purse. KeysPure ForceX Insect Repellant is my better smelling option.

Chapter 10

Traveling abroad and staying true to my new healthy diet

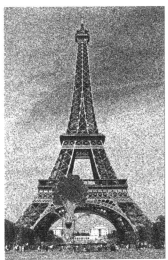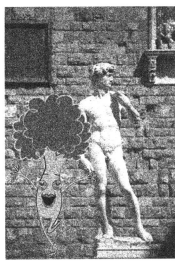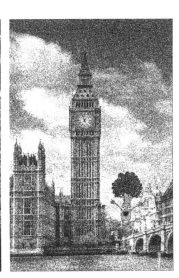

THE BIG TAKEAWAYS ON TRAVELING ABROAD AND STAYING TRUE TO MY NEW HEALTHY DIET:[61]

- *Travel takes planning. Yes, I know you plan for your flights and your rental car if you are flying, but you now also want to plan out how you will be healthy in your new location. I do this at least two weeks before I go anywhere.*

- *Whether or not you have sensitivities of your own that you avoid (see my chapter on sensitivities in my first book for a full explanation), or you have autoimmune disease, or you are a cancer survivor, or you have heart disease or even if you are healthy or a parent who wants to feed her children healthy food, understanding restaurants and how to eat out healthy is also important for you.*

- *Locate where the closest organic grocery stores are to buy healthy food before you book your hotel room. If you are going abroad, ask the hotel where you are staying for healthy food ideas.*

John and I have been to Europe twice in the five years since we married. We are not about to allow my autoimmune disease to hinder our enjoyment of life.

I will admit, in the beginning, I was nervous about how I was going to eat. It ended up being much easier than I would have thought.

The first time we went, we went to Italy for our honeymoon. We flew business class. I arranged for vegetarian food on the plane. And I hadn't learned yet to carry my emergency pack. So, dinner was difficult. It was soy-based, and soy is a sensitivity for me, but I did have the two big organic apples and almond butter that I had put into my carry-on bag, and they were a Godsend. I could eat the salad, just not the dressing. And not eating everything in sight was not terrible. I ate the nuts, and I decided I could eat the appetizer. Note to self: *don't order Vegan as it is heavily soy-based, and soy is a sensitivity*. Soy is also 95% GMO.

Since we were in business class (I used miles from all my years of travel), the stewards tried hard to accommodate me on both flights in both directions. They had an extra regular meal each direction, so they pulled the things off those meals that I could eat. I hadn't printed my sensitivity card yet, so I was listing what I couldn't eat from memory, and that made it somewhat confusing, but all in all, I got enough to eat at both meals.

I would have been better off not ordering a special meal, but I got the best of both worlds, so I was a lucky girl, and it worked out.

Once we got to Italy, I was fine. I discovered that although I thought I was sensitive to gluten, I was not. In the states, I was reacting to the Glyphosate, not to the gluten. (Right before harvesting the wheat, the wheat is drenched in Roundup, which shocks the plant and gives the farmer a larger harvest. The herbicide stays on the wheat through processing and is on all our wheat flours, crackers, pasta, bread, processed foods, etc. that aren't organic.) I am very sensitive to Glyphosate, which ends up being a blessing. Monsanto/Bayer has now lost three multimillion-dollar lawsuits against Glyphosate because it is known to cause cancer. Monsanto has known for 20 years that this herbicide causes cancer. There are now over 40,000 additional lawsuits pending. But the product is still being widely used on our food. I now eat organic wheat products, or I don't eat the item at all. Finding organic bread and pasta is becoming easier.) And in Italy, it was standard fare to get organic, unsprayed wheat products.

We went to Cinque Terra, which is part of the Italian Riviera, so fresh fish was easy to get, farm-fresh pastured eggs were easy, and since I wasn't reacting to the bread or the pasta and could eat them, I was home free. We went in March, so there were plenty of vegetables and fruits available.

We arrived in Italy one week before the tourist season. Ends up, that was the perfect time to go. The owners of the restaurant came and joined us at our meals, and since they weren't crazy busy, they were more than willing to cook for me. They bent over backward to accommodate me and to make me happy.

We discovered something interesting about the menus in Cinque Terra, and it ended up, it was consistent with the menus all over Italy. They all had a page in the back of their menu with 30 allergies and a number. When you read the menu, you would see the little numbers at the end of each dish. Instead of me needing to make a waiter run back and forth to the kitchen, asking whether a dish had certain ingredients, I could check for myself. How fantastic. If there was a dish, I was interested in that had, let's say, butter, now I could ask the waiter to ask the chef if he could make the dish with olive oil instead of the butter.

The list at the back of the Cinque Terra menus was very comprehensive. There was even a code for celery. Thank goodness, celery was not an issue for me. Ha!

When we asked the waiters or owners about the list, they commented that so many tourists had food sensitivities, it just made it easier for them. (I asked if it was only Americans, and they said no, lots of people from different places were suffering the same way that I was.) I loved that this list was at the back of all the menus because I could be responsible for what I was ordering right from the beginning. I wish that we used this system here in the USA. (We have shared this with many owners, so hopefully, someday. *smile*)

I had downloaded the Kindle version of the Rick Steves' Italy book, and it had a great section on all five towns in the Cinque Terra. Rick Steves (the PBS travel guide) adores Cinque Terra and goes there often. We used his guidebook as our guide to find food each day. Every day was an adventure but using the numbering system on the Italian menus made it easier for me to order.

Cinque Terra is five little towns in a row on the Italian Riviera. They are between Genoa and Pisa on the western Italian coast. The towns were all connected three ways, by train, by trail, and in-season by boat. Since we were there one week before the season began, we traveled and explored by train. The trails had glorious views, but the trails were uneven, and I was worried that I might not get good footage.

Cinque Terra is visually magnificent. The five towns were built in 1000 and were there to protect the coastline from invading pirates. In the 1500s, they protected the Italian coast against Turkish invaders. They started as fishing villages, and each home was painted a different pastel color. This way, it was easy for the fisherman to spot his home from the water. These colors have been maintained, and for me, made staying there a happy experience. The pastel colors spoke to me. There are grapevines for wine growing on the higher hillsides. Spectacular.

Since I was now relaxed about food, I was adventurous to explore.

We stayed in Vernazza overlooking the harbor. There were several seafood restaurants right on the waterfront right below our darling room, so our first nights, we ate there. We walked the entire town, and that included up the hill. There was a charming restaurant at the top of the village that Rick Steves had mentioned as a must, run by two brothers who were delightful (and the town comedians), so that's where we went for breakfast. I still thought that I was gluten sensitive at this point, and they were more than happy to accommodate me with some special pastries that they had just for customers like me. After I let them know what I was sensitive to, I let the brothers surprise me, and I got some very thinly cut meat with my pastry. Whatever it was, it was yummy. They don't serve eggs, but the rest of their offering was superb.

There was a restaurant in town that did serve eggs, The Blue Marlin. We went there the next morning. It had an American menu. The owner was delightful and had lived his whole life in Vernazza. He had hoped that his daughter would grow up and run his establishment, but she had chosen to go to school in the US and then to stay. He sat and told us stories of what it was like to grow up in Vernazza and to cook for generations of tourists. John and I were charmed, and the food was wonderful.

By the third day, I ventured to pasta. I was surprised that I did not react hostilely to it, and then my food choices opened up. I ate the bread; I ate the pasta; I had all the Italian favorites. And the toxins weren't in them, so my body was happy.

We visited other towns in the Cinque Terra and again followed the Rick Steves' suggestions. At one point, we sat in a large courtyard and ordered the recommended soup. Again, the owner joined us to share stories. We watched all the people on the street interact with each other and then cross the courtyard to interact with the restaurant's owner. The community was friendly and welcoming. The food was fabulous. The history of the buildings was all spelled out in the tour book. We fell in love with the place.

It was time to say "Ciao" and leave, so we grabbed the train to Florence. We stayed in a spectacular villa a little out of town up on the hill over the city, and the food within the hotel was incredible unto itself. Again, the menus all noted where the sensitivities in their dishes were. The hotel car would take us into Florence each day and drop us off close to the churches and museums that we wanted to see. We walked the city and found many a produce market tucked into nooks and crannies. Sometimes we would pick a restaurant randomly on the street, and other times, we returned to our hotel to enjoy their restaurants. Twice, we ventured back into Florence for dinner. The first time, I wanted a regular restaurant with locals. John found a family-run restaurant where mama was doing the accounting behind a counter in the back, papa was washing the wine glasses, and the two sons were serving us dinner. I don't remember what I ate, but it was a recipe that had been in their family for generations, and it was delicious. John had tripe, which is the famous dish of Tuscany.

The other night we found a young and very hip restaurant. I think we raised the median age in the restaurant by dozens of years. We had made a reservation, and I think they were a little confused that we wanted to eat there. It was a much fresher, modern take on Italian food. The restaurant was busy and noisy and the perfect opposite of the other restaurants we had eaten at up to that point. All the wait people in the restaurant were stopping by to chat with us about the US. It was loud and vibrant there, and we had a great time, and the food was marvelous.

Our final stop on this trip was to one of the grandest hotels on Lake Como. After all, it was our honeymoon.

First, our train was late, so we missed the boat that would take us around the lake to our hotel. We talked to the information person at the train station, and he recommended that we have Chinese food close to the bus stop and to wait for the bus there.

This was especially funny to me because years ago, my retail friends had taken an excursion to Lake Como after a buying trip. Their joke was that the one thing that this area needed was a Chinese restaurant. They weren't the only ones because now there was a Chinese restaurant in the perfect spot to get traffic. I stuck with vegetables and rice, and all was well.

One of our funniest stories about our honeymoon was about our wild hare bus ride halfway around the Lake. What the train guide had failed to mention was that the reason this bus was coming was to take all the school kids up the Lake to their homes since it was Friday. The bus was packed. I got on the bus in the front, but John got waved by the driver to enter from the back door. We were lugging all our luggage, I had half of it, and there was no place to sit, so I slowly scooted the luggage towards the back of the bus. The roads were narrow, and I could see over the cliffs to the water, and it felt rather harrowing. By the time I made it back to John, my husband asked me what stop we should get off at. Well, I hadn't thought to ask the driver as I was scooting my luggage on the floor, so I didn't have a clue.

A lovely well-dressed older Italian woman asked where we were going in broken English and then said we were to get off when she did. So, several stops down, she got off, so we got off too. No hotel was in sight. It was very windy, and we were standing by the edge of the cliff but had no idea where we were.

John called the hotel. He said we were stopped on Via Roma, and he gave them an address. The hotel said they had no clue where we were. We named off the businesses on the other side of the road, still confusion from the other end of the call. Suddenly John realized that he had called the hotel in Florence. Yikes. No wonder they didn't know how to retrieve us. (We were giggling a lot at this point, but still needed to find our hotel.)

So, John dug and found the phone number for our hotel. Yes, we were staying there that night, and we were two bus exits away. He would send the driver to come and get us.

When he arrived, the driver had an old woman in the car. She got out, and he unloaded all her groceries to the side of the road. She must have been 90. He was going to come back for her. He loaded all our luggage into the car, and then we got in.

The hotel we were staying at was spectacular. We gave the front desk our luggage and went to the porch restaurant overlooking the Lake for a quick bite. We were joined by another American couple who had just purchased a home right on the Lake; they were staying at our hotel while they purchased the furnishings. John commented that the homes on the Lake reminded him of Big Bear, CA, and the man's face fell. It put a bit of a halt in our conversation. Lake Como is one of the most exclusive locations in the world. Yikes. We were obviously not adequately impressed. (We have since gone to Big Bear, and I can see what my husband was referring to, but it's not remotely the same.)

The food in the restaurant was superb.

One note, when we checked in to our room, the hotel had reserved a newly remodeled room for us. The out-gassing from the paint and the new carpeting was overwhelming. There was no way that I could stay in that room. The gasses were toxic, especially harmful to my impaired immune system. We called the front desk, were very respectful but firm, and got moved to an older part of the hotel. Problem solved.

The restaurant in this hotel was staffed by men who had been on cruise lines. John had been on cruises dozens of times with his first wife, so they all bonded with us. They, too, had the page with all the sensitivities on the last page of their menu. They made a note of what I could eat, and after the first day, as soon as we sat down, they would bring foods to munch on while we decided what we wanted for our main courses, and they always had recommendations of what I could eat.

In other words, my first trip to Europe after getting an autoimmune disease and discovering my 15 sensitivities was a gastronomical delight. Their food system has not been corrupted as ours has, and it was very easy for me to find delicious, non-toxic live foods that made my body happy. I ate healthily, and around all my food sensitivities, I didn't have a flare that would have caused pain, so all was well.

Flash forward two years, and John and I returned to Europe, but this time, first to England and then to France.

We stayed in a darling boutique hotel in London, just down the street from Harrods, which made the old retailer in me happy as a clam. I was going to do my first podcast about my book while I was in London, so I had brought a copy of the book to give to the show host. Unfortunately, an elder parent of the show host fell, so we didn't get to do the interview. In chatting with the woman staffing the front desk, I discovered that she had just become a Mom. I offered her my book to read. She was speed reading it the rest of the time we were in the hotel so that she could pass it on to other support crew there. They were all so excited by my book, (**It Feels Good to Feel Good, Learn to Eliminate Toxins, Reduce Inflammation and Feel Great Again**) it made my heart warm.

We had chatted extensively with the hotel staff about my need for toxin-free food, so they started doing research. By now, I had all my sensitivities on a business card, so I had given them copies. Breakfast was easy once again because the pastries were made with organic flour. We had eggs and veggies, and all were delicious. We went to one of the museums during the day. Then we walked Harrods (a famous department store in London) before we returned to our hotel that night. If we needed it, Harrods had a food emporium for us to return to. The hotel staff had found a perfect restaurant to recommend to us for dinner, and it was only a few blocks away.

This restaurant did not have a system like Italy. However, they did have a special menu for folks with sensitivities, so they were very easy to work with, and I had a delicious dinner.

The next day we took the bus tour all around London after we repeated our scrumptious breakfast. When we got back to our hotel, we decided to have High Tea. It was a little tricky finding things on the menu that I could eat, but I had brought a jar of ghee with me, which I went up and got, and the chef then made me little finger sandwiches with ham and ghee and cucumber and also a variety of roasted vegetable sandwiches. Because they made all my sandwiches just for me, I got enough to serve an army, so they put the extra in a cute little box so that I could take them up to the room for the next day's tea.

I looked on Google for "tea" in London and discovered there are several restaurants that serve a variety of teas, including one that is Vegan. There is also a London bus tour that serves tea, and a vegan tea is available. Do your research before you go. The world is your oyster if you plan.

John had hired a driver to take us to Bath and Stonehenge on our third day in London. Our driver was a retired copper who had majored in history and was exceptionally knowledgeable about the areas we went through on our trip. The restaurant we ate in for lunch in Bath was the only iffy choice of our trip, but we found something for me to eat, and all was well, and I had my little tea sandwiches to eat the minute we returned to our hotel, so all was well. We picked food out at the Harrods deli for that night, and what they have to offer was amazing—a true gourmet delight.

Then we jumped on the train to Paris.

In France, I was in food heaven. All fresh ingredients. All pastured meat. All toxin-free fish. Who knew it would be so easy to eat in France?

We were meeting my ex-sister-in-law (still a dear friend) and her husband in central France. They bought a home there a few years ago, and we were delighted to have an opportunity to explore France with friends who knew the terrain.

I printed my sensitivities card in French. My friends thought that I had lost my mind, and the French would never work around my food peculiarities. The French took tremendous pride in what they prepared for their meals, and my friends did not think that they would work around my idiosyncrasies.

So, we take the train to central France and our friends fetched us from the train station and took us directly to the hotel we were all staying in that night. They had arranged for us to have dinner that night in a troglodyte restaurant. Part of the walls were ancient caves that people had lived in hundreds of years previously. The restaurant was fascinating.

I don't speak French, but I pulled out my card and gave it to the waiter. Everyone grimaced. The waiter smiled at me and came around the table and patted me on my shoulder. "Oh, Madam, I am so sorry," he said in broken English. "Not to worry, I will make you something fabulous." And he did. My meal was amazing. Everyone was jealous. And from then on, I knew I was home free in France.

The French cook with fresh organic vegetables and with grass-fed meats and wild fish. They take great pride in using only the finest ingredients. Since they cook from scratch, it was not inconvenient for them to work around and leave out the ingredients I couldn't eat. And my food was fantastic.

They even have a thing about not asking for a doggy bag. They feel that it would reduce the quality of their food too much to take it home for a different meal. (It was almost like an insult.)

I only had one iffy meal while we were in France. It was at a tourist spot where an old Roman monument to Mercury was being excavated at the top of a mountain, Puy de Dome, in the Auvergne region of France. We had lunch at the monument. I think in the end, I got a salad. I made it work. By now, I had my emergency pack, so that tided me over to the next meal.

One of our highlights was to go to the residence of da Vinci[62] in the last years of his life. da Vinci was a vegetarian, and they have maintained his gardens, and they had some of his inventions displayed in miniature and in full size on the property. This was where da Vinci finished the Mona Lisa, which is why it is in the Louvre instead of in an Italian Museum. It was down the hill from a French King who offered him the home and built a tunnel from the castle to da Vinci's kitchen. There, they would sit together and have stimulating intellectual conversations on the state of the world.

There was a charming garden restaurant at this tourist location, and the food was first class. It was easy for me to order and eat. It was one of the highlights of our visit.

We also visited the home of Catherine de' Medici. She was a very powerful woman and the mother of 5 French kings/queens. Her home also became very important during WWII since the line between Nazi territory and Vichy territory went right through the castle, so some refugees were able to escape by going through the castle.

The most interesting meal that we had was at a restaurant that only offered one entrée each night. We sat out on a patio and watched the world go by. The entrée of the evening was pigeon. (my sister in laws husband, went yuk when the owner left our table), but what the heck, when in France, eat like the French. It tasted like chicken and was quite tasty.

I remember years ago when I went to Rome on a buying trip with my boss in the jewelry industry; we were invited to the home of a friend of hers who served sparrow. The little feet were sticking up. They were delicious, but a little harder to handle psychologically.

The little feet were also sticking out on the pigeon legs. Our friend took the breast pieces (unidentifiable), whereas my hubby, John, was more than delighted to eat the legs with the feet. (John will eat anything, I swear. *smile*) My sister-in-law and I ate both types of pieces.

We visited many of the castles of central France and then went to spend a few nights at our friend's home. We got to see how they shopped and the high quality of fruits and veggies in the area. Susan and I had fun cooking together. It was lovely to be back in a kitchen and cooking again.

I will admit I was a bit of a glutton with the bread and pastries that were available in the area. The only organic bread that we had found in Los Angeles at the time was Sourdough from our farmer's market. There were amazing types of bread, croissants, and other pastries available that I could eat in France, and I thoroughly enjoyed all of them, sometimes several at a time. Aarrgghh. I was in food heaven.

From here, John and I jumped on the train and went back to Paris. We walked the Champs-Élysées and enjoyed looking at all the historic buildings and where Thomas Jefferson had lived. There was another famous restaurant where all the authors from the 1920s used to eat and drink—famous writers like Scott Fitzgerald, and Hemmingway, and artists like Monet and Picasso. As we walked, we read menus and made notes as to where we wanted to dine.

Food did not disappoint. We had two unique experiences that I want to share.

We went to the Louvre and spent a day (and saw the real Mona Lisa), and as we were leaving, we decided to get a bicycle cab. Our driver was a lovely young woman from Romania. She had worked for Tony Robbins at one point in Italy, so we immediately bonded. We then decided we would call her the next day to take us to Notre Dame.

She knew a restaurant across the street from the cathedral. She took us by the restaurant on our way to Notre Dame and introduced us to the owner. She explained to him how I needed to eat. We then continued our sightseeing. The restaurant owner then went to the market to prepare a special meal for us, and we headed back there for dinner. He made me his favorite vegetable soup and a special fish. The restaurant was old and went back, I think, to the 15th century. It was an amazing spot and a fabulous meal.

We then called Roxy (our cab driver) the next day because she had another spot to show us for dinner. She dropped us off in an upscale Millennial hamburger joint. It was amazing. The owner had gotten each of the famous chefs of the French Cooking tv show to design a special hamburger for her restaurant. John had a squid ink bun with a fish burger; I had a grass-fed burger on a homemade organic bun. This restaurant owner was so committed to health, she made her ketchup, mustard, and bottled her filtered water in glass containers. We had organic French fries that were cooked in rice bran oil and covered with sea salt. The restaurant was small, but we got to chat with the owner, and we had a fabulous time.

The food in our hotel was also delicious, and we had breakfast there every morning and dinner in their dining room once. The other nights we picked from the restaurants we had spotted as we walked the Champs-Élysées. We walked the streets and visited the Paris farmers' markets. We chatted with the local Parisians. Food wasn't an issue, and our trip was wonderful.

My final observation about where we traveled in Europe.

Our experience in Italy and France was that they use fresh local ingredients whenever possible. They are not serving processed food or food in baggies that are microwaved and rearranged, as they now do in many American restaurants. Our eating in England was more limited, so I don't know if that observation is across the board in England, but our hotel found us wonderful restaurants that used fresh ingredients and cooked around my sensitivities.

- My key point once again is, don't be shy. Ask for what you need.
- Our motto is to be flexible, be forceful, and be grateful.
- Don't be an ugly American. I have traveled extensively to Asia. I have encountered plenty of obnoxious Americans. There is just no excuse for it. One was screaming at the front desk of a high-end hotel, "How stupid are you! Can't you speak English?". I calmly and quietly said behind him, "How about you speak Thai." (and got 'the glare') I have found that people everywhere, especially in hospitality, want to help you. Be kind and give them that opportunity.
- Be as charming as possible. People in Europe tried hard to make me happy and get me what I needed. And they went out of their way for me. If you have a health issue, tell them that. I was not the only customer that had made such requests. If you don't have a health issue, tell them that anyway, and get clean food.

One comment on traveling to Asia in earlier years.

I went there before I was aware of ingredients or toxins and sensitivities. However, I am a complete spice wuss. Ends up, I don't only dislike hot spices; they dramatically impact my body negatively. We went to lunch in a restaurant where I got to choose a fresh fish and then all the veggies that I wanted to have cooked with it. Brilliant. However, the Thai put hot red peppers in everything, and they use hot red pepper oil. As I took my first bite, I bit into a hot red pepper. I didn't know what to do with it, so I held it in my mouth. My business partner grabbed my arm and said, spit it out. I didn't want to be rude, and I didn't want to do that. My entire face turned bright red, and it started down my neck and chest. I finally spit it out. Everyone at the table was horrified. Once the crisis was over, we all laughed.

I had a Thai friend write a list with two columns with what I wanted to eat for breakfast, lunch, and dinner. One side was in English; the other side was in Thai. I could point to what I wanted, and the waiter could see what it was. The top of the paper said something like. No hot red peppers. Zero, none. No hot red oil floating on top. Take it out. If you can't, do not let me order it. Worked like a charm. They would laugh, but they would bring me food without the heat. Speak up for what you need, no matter what the situation. People will help you.

The woman at the front desk in London, who I gave my book to, was amazed that we didn't know what items have GMOs that we buy in the US. They have truth in labeling in the UK. They warned us that if we went to Spain, Spain was growing GMO crops, so buyer beware.

The food we found and the people we met made for an extraordinary experience in Europe. Having friends that we adore that were familiar to France made for a perfect vacation and enhanced our experience. I look forward to a return trip.

> Note—Be careful when coming back to the USA. There is a program called "Don't Pack a Pest." You are not allowed to bring many agricultural products into the country from overseas. It does not seem to matter where the fruit originated from. If you forget to eat it or leave it on the plane, please declare it to the appropriate agent. Do not throw it out in the Airport.

Chapter 11

Keys to taking a cruise and maintaining a "clean," healthy lifestyle

A guest chapter by John Gins, my husband

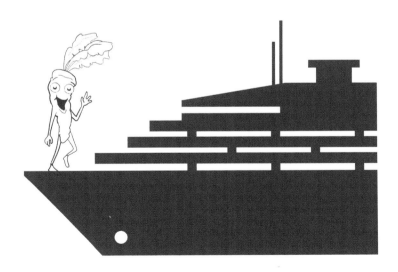

THE BIG TAKEAWAYS ON TAKING A CRUISE AND MAINTAINING A "CLEAN" HEALTHY LIFESTYLE:[63]

- *Travel takes planning.*
- *If the chef is not accommodating what you need to eat, speak up, and be firm, but always treat the workers on the cruise with respect.*

From Cheryl -

I don't cruise for a couple of reasons. First of all, I get claustrophobic on the boat, which would be a bit of a problem when I was out on the ocean, and secondly, I like to go, travel, interact with the people in the part of the world that I am visiting, get to "feel" the culture, get to "see" the country, and to go with the flow.

My husband, John, took ten cruises with his wife of forty-two years. They saw the world this way and loved it.

Not to diminish John's previous travel experiences, I was happy to introduce him to my way of travel. I have traveled extensively for the jewelry business.

John and I have now had fun adventures a result. It also has given John a different perspective, which I think is a good thing (a new wife, new experiences.)

John lost his first wife of 43 years to cancer shortly before we met. He was devastated. When we met, he had already booked himself on a trip around the world, and I encouraged him to go. I believed that he needed to know who he was alone if we were going to stand a chance as a couple. His trip was 90 days.

These are his observations from his many years of cruising, and he offered to share his experiences with my readers. When he took his last cruise, he had already converted to a healthy lifestyle.

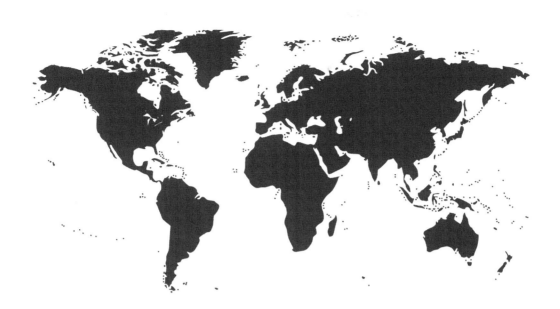

This is what John wrote:

I joke that my first cruise was in 1965 when I was a Marine on a troop carrier going from San Diego to Okinawa en route to Vietnam.

This troop carrier held 3000 of us; we were passengers living in confined spaces. The bunks were stacked about four hammocks high. This was not a luxurious cruise.

We pretty much lived between meals; we got in line for breakfast, lunch, and dinner. We got in line for the restrooms or as we called it the head. We got in line for just about everything, so it was anything but an interesting experience. However, I did experience a typhoon during that trip. It was a bit unnerving.

Fast forward to being married to my first wife. My wife Margie and I decided to take a cruise around Hawaii for our 25th anniversary.

Margie and I prepared for this cruise by taking a shorter 4-day cruise to Ensenada, to make sure that we would be able to take an ocean voyage. I wasn't worried about getting seasick, but Margie was not sure. We enjoyed the cruising itself, but we were not that crazy about the social scene on the ship. There was a very young crowd on this cruise.

For our next trip, we flew to Hawaii and took a seven-day cruise around the Hawaiian Islands. We got to visit places we would not have seen if we had just flown into Oahu. We took the tours that were offered by the cruise, and we both had an excellent time. We did learn how to kayak, and we did this activity several times after we got back home. We got bit by the joy of cruising.

A couple of years later, we decided to take our children, ages 10 and 14 at the time, on a cruise to the Caribbean. We flew into San Juan, Puerto Rico, explored San Juan for several days, and then took a cruise around the Virgin Islands. I know that my children were quite impressed. Eric came back and did a lot of artwork reflecting the trip. The Montserrat volcano eruption occurred a year later, and Amy did a science project about that.

Finally, in 2000, we took our big trip with the children. We flew to England and took a cruise from Dover to Rome in August. I think, as a family, we were able to get a feel for what it was like to be outside of the US. We saw things that we had heard about, and now we were experiencing them firsthand.

I was not conscious of eating healthy in those days, but I was conscious of my weight. So, my principal form of exercise on a cruise was walking the deck. I entered the shipboard contests, and invariably, I would come in close to the top of the challenges.

In total, Margie and I took ten cruises over the years. We continued cruising after Margie was diagnosed with cancer. We went during the periods when she was feeling better. We went on a cruise of the Baltic and Russia. Iceland, Scotland, Ireland, and England were all fun places to visit. The Panama Canal during the latest construction phase was very interesting and insightful. I got a much better appreciation of how people live outside of the US.

I was not as health conscious as I am now, so we ate freely from the ship's offerings.

My last cruise in 2014 was a 90-day cruise around the world. I took this a year and a half after Margie died. I arranged my trip, and then I met Cheryl about two weeks later. Cheryl does not like to cruise, but she encouraged me to travel solo.

I was able to let the wind blow through my mind on this 90-day voyage.

I was now committed to healthy living and eating. I was diagnosed with diabetes earlier that year; by lowering my carbohydrate intake, I lost 80 pounds with Cheryl's help. I ended up going on this cruise after suffering from an almost fatal bleeding incident due to an allergic reaction to one of my medications. My doctors cleared me for the cruise, but they told me to avoid vigorous exercise. On every other cruise, I walked the decks to maintain my weight, so this concerned me.

Through my travel agent, I arranged that I would talk with the maître d' each evening to study the following day's menu. This routine was set up to help me determine what low carbohydrate food I would be able to eat the next day. Then the plan was that I could customize my meal. This plan did not work out during the first couple of days. I realized that I wasn't getting the chef's attention, and I could not find the correct person to help me. I called my travel agent from the ship and told her I needed help with food, or that I would need to leave the ship. My phone call got attention.

As a result, each morning, I was presented with the next day's menu. With my new knowledge of healthy food, I was able to stick to my low carbohydrate diet, and I could get exactly the food that I needed to eat. At times, it required me to find something on the menu that could be substituted to go with my main protein. If I couldn't make that work, I knew that I could go to one of the specialty restaurants. (We had a sushi restaurant on the ship that was easy to access.)

This trip helped me improve my socialization skills. This was the only advantage of traveling solo, which is difficult, especially for that long of a period. I was lonely. Halfway through the voyage, I decided to start getting massages. For every two weeks during the remainder of the cruise. I enjoyed the massage. I had forgotten how important it is to have physical contact and touch from somebody else. Then a group of older women adopted me. I joined their table and ate my meals with them. The ringleader was well into her 90's. As a result, I made several friends on the ship, and I now keep in touch with them.

One of the challenges on a moving ship is to figure out how to measure your weight. There are scales in the gym, but since the ship sways, the needle moves on the scale. I realized that what I had to do was let the needle go back-and-forth a couple of times and essentially take the average to get an estimate of what I weighed. Although this was not ideal, it was better than nothing. I made it work.

As we were all getting ready to dock in our last port, one of my friends said to me, "John, I don't know how you've kept your weight off; you didn't exercise. I've never seen you walking. How did you do it?" I told him I was very conscious of only eating low-carb foods, which was necessary to control my diabetes.

Bread is one of my big weaknesses, so early on the cruise, I told my waitpersons, "If you want a tip at the end of this cruise, stop offering me bread." They became very good about not tempting me with bread from that point forward. This was a very wise move on my part. They no longer tempted me with the bread, and this way, I could avoid eating it.

When I got off the ship and weighed myself at home, I was exactly the same weight as when I got on the ship. I was very pleased.

I learned the value of having massages on this trip. My gift to Cheryl, instead of bringing her knickknacks, has been for us to get couples massages every two weeks.

My final advice is to be a conscious traveler. Plan on how to provide yourself with healthy options; and be flexible about your expectations. Enjoy the changes that result from this type of experience. Try and place yourselves into other people's shoes. It was important for me to be firm about what I could eat on the ship to maintain my health. But I was always grateful for their assistance.

As Cheryl commented in her chapter about traveling in Europe, plan, but remain firm about what you can and cannot eat.

I was out of my comfort zone on this trip, but in the end, I had delicious, healthy food. I made new friends, and I saw some exceptional places around the globe.

When I got off the ship, I asked Cheryl to marry me.

I am editing this account six years after the cruise. I realized that this cruise experience was critical for my individual growth. I retired from my statistical career when I turned 70 in 2016. I realized that I was motivated to learn how to improve my health, expand my knowledge, and to give back to my community and the world. I have found that my purpose in life is to become a teacher—not necessarily a Mathematics Professor but of how to have a productive, healthy, and joyful life.

Cheryl and I have learned a lot together. I am delighted to partner with her in this endeavor.

John Gins, aka Chun Mok.[64]

Part V

Taking Care of You

Chapter 12

How to Keep Stress Levels Low Using a Series of Three Minute Exercises

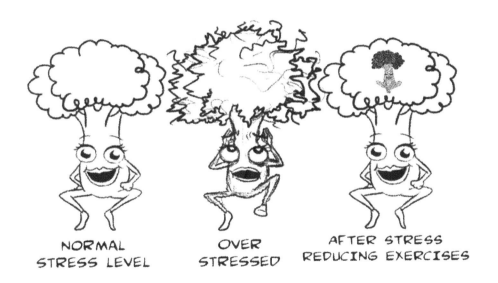

NORMAL STRESS LEVEL   OVER STRESSED   AFTER STRESS REDUCING EXERCISES

THE BIG TAKEAWAYS ON HOW TO KEEP STRESS LEVELS LOW USING A SERIES OF THREE MINUTE EXERCISES:[65]

- *95% of all illness is either caused by or worsened by stress.*

- *"If you knew what was happening to your body when you're stressed out, you would freak out." Mark Hyman, MD*

- *Chronic stress can affect every physical and psychological system. We all deal with stress as we go through our day. It's when it accumulates that it becomes an issue. It's important to release your stress every day so that it doesn't build up.*

- *Recovery is not negotiable; you can either make time to rest and rejuvenate now or make time to be sick and injured later.*

- *Some of the exercises below are breathing exercises. Others are small movement exercises. None of them take more than 3 minutes each. It's important to use them singularly throughout the day.*

This chapter is an update on everything I have learned about stress since I wrote my first book. I thought stress was helping me get more done in my jewelry business, so I thought I was thriving on stress. I never realized that stress was hindering my productivity and hurting my brain and slowing me down as a result. Once I got sick, I came to a screeching halt because of stress.

I believe this information is so important that I revised my chapter on stress in my first book[66] and am repeating the newest information here. 95% of all illness is either caused by or worsened by stress.[67] I want you to have access to these stress exercises no matter which of my books you pick up.

I had to learn ways to release my stress. My cortisol was almost to Addison's Disease when I got autoimmune disease eight years ago. This was a result of my body's reaction to the chronic stress that I had in my life.

*"If you knew what was happening to your body
when you're stressed out, you would freak out."*

MARK HYMAN, MD

Most chronic illnesses have stress as one of their core issues. Stress creates Leaky Gut, which is the root cause of chronic illness, and it wreaks havoc on all our major organs. I had to learn to get my stress under control, or I couldn't get well.

Chronic stress can affect every physical and psychological system. We all deal with stress as we go through our day. It's when it accumulates that it becomes an issue. It's important to release your stress every day so that it doesn't build up.

Chronic stress impacts the following:

- Heart Disease
- High Blood Pressure
- It breaks down the immune system and makes us susceptible to infection
- It contributes to "leaky gut," which leads to inflammation and pain. Stress releases inflammatory substances that travel through your body and attack body tissues. Stress causes disease.
- Stress causes muscles to tighten and contract.
- Over time stress creates back and neck pain and headaches
- Stress increases the permeability of the blood-brain barrier, allowing toxins, viruses, and poisons to flow through.
- Stress causes us to crave high-sugar, high-salt foods that release dopamine, a feel-good brain chemical that leads to more cravings.
- Stress causes increased sugar cravings. Sugar is a toxin, as addictive as cocaine, and it feeds cancer and causes inflammation. It turns off Ghrelin, a hormone that regulates appetite, and that makes you hungry.
- Stress messes with your memory and brain functions. Stress impacts mood, causing anxiety and depression.
- Stress causes weight gain and increased belly fat.
- Stress causes digestive issues.

- Stress reduces blood flow to the skin causing skin disorders (Psoriasis, Eczema, acne)

Finding ways to reframe stress in our lives is crucial for reversing inflammation and squelching the degeneration of our tissues and the diseases of aging. Powerful stuff.

Recovery is not negotiable; you can either make time to rest and rejuvenate now or make time to be sick and injured later.

The long-term activation of the stress-response system and the overexposure to cortisol and other stress hormones that follow can disrupt almost all your body's processes. This puts you at increased risk of many health problems, including:

Anxiety
Depression
Digestive problems
Headaches
Heart disease
Sleep problems
Weight gain
Memory and concentration impairment
Leaky gut and autoimmune disease

I discussed stress at length in my first book, but since I published it, I have found and implemented several stress exercises into my daily regime. These are a series of short exercises. Most of them take no equipment, and most do not take longer than 2 to 3 minutes each. But each of these exercises releases whatever stress has accumulated in your body, and also, they send energy to the brain, improving productivity.

The first breathing exercise is one I have now been utilizing since I first got sick. This is the 4-7-8 breathing exercise by Andrew Weil, MD, the first Integrative doctor. You can google him and do the exercise with him on YouTube.

I use this exercise when I feel frustration or stress coming on. I use this exercise when I am having a hard time going to sleep at night. I use this exercise in LA traffic when I realize I could be late for an appointment, and there is nothing I can do about it. In most cases, no one around me even knows I am doing it. It immediately calms me and resets my parasympathetic nervous system.

I know how well this breathing exercise works because I use it when I am driving through LA traffic at rush hour to a functional MD appointment 1 hour away from my home. I hate it when my blood pressure is high, and my pulse is also reflecting the stress of my drive when I get to my MD office and get monitored. Since I have started using this exercise, my blood pressure is within an appropriate range, and my pulse is lower than most patients that my MD sees.

It works.

But beyond this, I now have a whole routine that I practice. This entire set of exercises is what I recommend to you.

BEFORE YOU RISE

- Stretch from the tips of your fingers to the tips of your toes
- Take three deep breathes
- Do a fast palm rub with your hands over your chest close to your body. Do this for 30 seconds
- Do the spinal twist. Bring your knees to your chest, and then take one leg across your other leg and twist your back. Put your arms into a cactus position and turn your head in the opposite direction. Switch.

WHEN YOU FIRST GET OUT OF BED

- Stand up slowly and touch your toes. Hold it for 5 seconds
- Now, standing, raise your arms above your head to touch the ceiling. Hold it for 5 seconds
- Stretch your neck to the right and hold it for 5 seconds
- Turn your head to the right and hold it for 5 seconds
- Turn your head to the left and hold it for 5 seconds.

MORNING

- **Greet the Sunrise—This could be as simple as looking out a window to view the Sunrise** and expressing gratitude. Sunrise is my favorite part of the day, and its spectacularly different every morning.
- You could also do the yoga routine to salute the sun.[68]

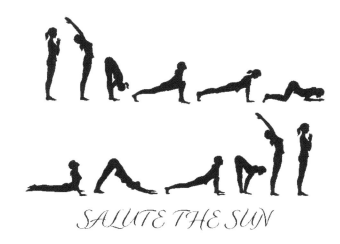

SALUTE THE SUN

- Morning papers-[69] "Morning Pages are three pages of longhand, a stream of consciousness writing, done first thing in the morning. There is no wrong way to do Morning Pages. They are not high art. They are not even "writing." They are for your eyes only. Morning Pages provoke, clarify, comfort, cajole, prioritize, and synchronize the day at hand. Do not over-think Morning Pages: just put three pages of anything on the page and then do three more pages tomorrow." These are "cloud-thoughts." "You are meeting your shadow and taking it out for a cup of coffee." It's a great way to clear out your "dark thoughts" before you start your day.
- Morning pages are also a great way to uncover deep-seated creativity.
- Take additional Magnesium, which relaxes the body. It is common nowadays to have a magnesium deficiency. Magnesium is considered the relaxation mineral.

Most importantly, list five things you are grateful for that morning. This allows you to start your day on a very positive note. It keeps you in the now and erases past negativity.

Stress builds up all day long. Every hour, take 1-3 minutes to release the buildup by using these methods:

- Dr. Weil's 4-7-8 breathing exercise 4 rounds at least 2x daily. This resets your parasympathetic nervous system. (Look it up on YouTube and do it with him.)[70]
- Take your fingers and push into your belly button and jiggle for 1 minute. The theory is that your belly button is the beginning of our life, and through our belly button, we can impact the entire body.[71]
- If you are in a private space, use the Belly Button Wand.[72] But if you are in a public space, your fingers work just fine. This affects your reptilian brain at the back of your neck (the early brain in development) and significantly reduces your stress as proven by Dr. Emerel Mayer, executive director of the Oppenheimer Center for Stress and Resilience (uclacns.org) and the Co-director of the Digestive Diseases Research Center at the University of California at Los Angeles. (see my comment later in this chapter.)
- Stand and bounce in place every hour to break up the day. This will bring energy to the brain. Stand up by your desk, let your arms hang, and bounce. Do this for 1-2 minutes.
- Tapping the body starting at the ankles and working up to the top of the head. Don't hurry. Do front and back of your feet, your ankles. As you do these, do up one side and down the other. Do your calves, your thighs, your tummy, your heart zone, go over to your arm and start with one hand and tap all the way up, and then all the way down, then do the other, now tap your shoulders, your face and then the top of your head. This should take 2 minutes.
- Every hour on the half-hour, stretch at your desk. Be sure to stretch up and stretch out. You can do it seated, or you can stand.
- I just learned a new stress releaser that you do from a sitting position. Put your hands on the side of your thighs (at the same time, one hand

on the outside of each thigh) push out to build resistance. Hold for 10 seconds and release. You will feel relaxation go through your entire body.
- Then do the opposite, put your hands on the inside of your thighs and build resistance by pushing in against your hands.
- When fatigued, toe-tap from a sitting position. Just put your legs out straight and tap your toes.
- Rest Your Eyes and Turn Off the Lights

The Belly Button Wand is an excellent tool to release stress.[73]

"Eastern medicine has known for thousands of years the importance of the belly button as an acupressure point. The belly button was even used as a stimulating point to revive someone in emergency treatment when a person suddenly lost consciousness or has collapsed due to high blood pressure or stroke!

In Eastern medicine, the acupressure point in the belly button is known as "Shin-gwol," which means "the place where God resides." The belly button is the place where life starts and is received and transferred by the embryo via the umbilical cord in its mother's womb. Your belly button is not just a scar left over from birth! It is a very important acupressure point in recovering health and vitality."

Increasing Blood Circulation

A fascinating study reported by the Los Angeles Times and The Washington Post shows the effectiveness of stimulating the abdomen. Researchers from the St. Joseph's Hospital and Medical Center in Paterson, NJ, provided treatment for resuscitating 103 emergency patients whose breathing was gradually stopping. There were two kinds of treatment: one was the conventional method of CPR on the chest; the other was a method that involved abdominal compressions in addition to traditional CPR. Amazingly, the recovery rate with the chest-CPR was no more than 7%, while the recovery rate with the abdominal compressions was more than triple that of only the chest at a surprising 25%.

- So how does it work? Your gut holds one-third of your entire body's blood supply. When we put pumping pressure on the abdomen through Belly Button Healing, it circulates the blood collected around your vital organs throughout the entire body from head to toe. Regular blood circulation is the key to revitalized energy.
- When you lack vitality or are feeling the afternoon slump, pressing on the belly button using Belly Button Healing can help your body recover vigor and warmth.

The Belly Button Wand was introduced to us in our Body and Brain Yoga classes. We now stay up to date with the teachings of Ilchi Lee, who is the Master of the organization. We have learned a multitude of ways to improve our stress levels, our mindset, and our health from this group. One of the reasons we bought our second home in Sedona is because we went a few times to their 150-acre retreat Mago in Sedona, which is amazingly beautiful, and we fell in love with the area.

My husband and I often use the belly button wand on each other. We lay on the floor and take turns. It is a very loving thing to do for each other, and it releases my stress.

I want to tell you the story of the first time we met Dr. Emerel Mayer at UCLA. We had gone to a presentation, and Ilchi Lee was there to give him a Belly Button Wand. Dr. Meyer had his brain electrode machine set up, and initially, he poo-pooed the wand. But he pulled a few people out of the crowd to prove that the wand would not work. They took a reading which had erratic brain waves, and then they handed the subject a belly button wand and showed him how to use it for 2 minutes. They then took a second reading. The lines were much calmer and much less erratic. Dr. Mayer became a fan.

We ran into Dr. Mayer again at a Health Fair in the San Fernando Valley, and we got into a conversation with him about his surprise that the wand worked as well as it did.

John bought me an aura machine for my birthday. I had commented in passing that I would love to have one, and he wants to make me happy, so he bought it for me. We often do readings when we go to health fairs. John takes the readings for the client. It is a great tool to read the body's energy and see where the body is out of order, and then I give health advice about how to get back into balance. We take two readings for each person. One before using the belly button wand, and one after. They are usually night and day. It's fascinating. We did one woman at a health fair last fall, and her energy was originally all shades of grey. She then used the belly button wand and regained some color in her aura. Ends up, she was recovering from a severe chronic illness and operation. It's a fantastic tool for health and for releasing stress.

The benefits of breaking up your day with mini stress releasing exercises:

- You send blood to your brain, release the stress, and relax.
- You also wake your body up to feel alive.
- You will think better and be more productive.
- You will improve your digestion and reduce the possibility of inflammation.

You will significantly lower your stress.

You eliminate the possibility of your stress building up to a chronic level by letting off steam throughout the day. This is incredibly good for your long-term health.

The world needs you at your best.

You are at your best when you resonate with your soul and focus inwardly on your heart. You are at your best when you are in balance and fully present in your life. You are at your best when your stress is low, and your brain is clear. These exercises will allow you to achieve that. Start them today.

Stop overcommitting yourself. It's ok to take care of you, and to say NO!

"You have to learn to say no without feeling guilty. Setting boundaries is healthy. You need to learn to respect and take care of yourself."

UNKNOWN AWESOMEQUOTES4U.COM

Note—This is becoming one of the most popular subjects that I am asked to speak about. Stress is a universal issue, and learning these releases is so important for all of us in this busy world.

Chapter 13

The Benefits of Gratitude

Cheryl's Gratitude Board

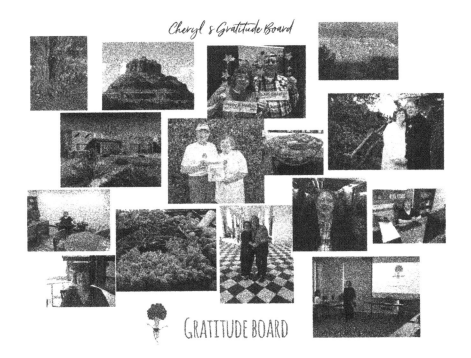

GRATITUDE BOARD

THE BIG TAKEAWAYS ON THE BENEFITS OF GRATITUDE:[74]

- *Grateful Living is a way of life that asks us to notice everything in our lives that is present and abundant—from the littlest things of beauty to the grandest of our blessings—so that we do not take anything for granted.*

- *Giving thanks sets the mood for the entire day has a lasting effect on your mood.*

- *Gratitude allows you to see setbacks as challenges you can get past. There is joy in figuring out how to accomplish challenges, and as you get over the hurdle, they then enhance your life.*

It is a given that all of us, no matter where we are in the world, want to be happy.

We need to stop, get quiet, take a moment, to open our eyes and our senses to everything around us that is good, to foster happiness.

Grateful Living is a way of life that asks us to notice everything in our lives that is present and abundant—from the littlest things of beauty to the grandest of our blessings—to that we do not take anything for granted.

"What is gratitude? It's an affirmation of goodness, that life is good and rewarding, and that goodness comes from outside of ourselves. We affirm that there are good things in the world, gifts, and benefits we've received."

"Grateful Living is supported by daily practices, tools, habits of mind, and behaviors that can be learned, translated, and applied to many aspects of our lives. It is nourished in community and relationships.

Being grateful every day can uplift us, make a difference for others, and help change the world.

We acknowledge that other people—and even a higher power if you're a spiritual person—bless us with gifts that bring the goodness in our lives."

"I see it as a relationship-strengthening emotion." Writes Emmons, the leading expert on gratitude, "Because it requires us to see how we've been supported and affirmed by other people."[75]

Being grateful starts with an acknowledgment of what in our lives is enjoyable and rewarding.

Just getting up and saying, "It's great to be alive" is an excellent place to start.

Practicing gratitude encourages a person to stop and acknowledge loved ones, colleagues, animals, and, of course, mother nature. Gratitude also allows us to stop and make amends or solve issues in the now. Feeling gratitude does not require reciprocity from anyone else, which has a karmic quality in and of itself. It merely allows the receiver to pay the goodness forward, generating more positivity.

GRATITUDE PROMOTES GRATITUDE.

All spiritual practices encourage us to stay in the now and reflect on our blessings.

Gratitude multiplies our joy as many times as we "stop, look, and pay attention!"

Characteristics of grateful people:

- You feel a sense of abundance in your life.
- You appreciate and acknowledge the contributions others have made to your well-being.
- You recognize and enjoy life's little pleasures.
- You acknowledge the importance of experiencing and expressing gratitude. That, in itself, makes you happy.
- You are more resilient and bounce back from tough emotions.

- Gratitude encourages you to take nothing for granted.
- It allows you to celebrate the present.
- It enables you to participate in the good things in your life instead of just being a spectator. It allows you to stop and take notice.
- Gratitude blocks negative emotions, envy, regret, resentment, and depression. New studies show that it reduces depression.
- It allows you to see the rainbow in every cloud.
- Being grateful reduces your suffering, and it reduces anxiety, at the same time as motivating positive emotions.
- You stop taking things and people for granted, and you take the time to reflect on their contributions to your life, which strengthens your social connections.

Giving thanks has a lasting effect on your mood and sets the mood for the entire day. There is a gift in everything, even challenges. The point is to find and focus on that gift to set your mood.

The key is to find the positive in seemingly bad situations and not to miss the other good things going on around you.

Gratitude allows you to see setbacks as challenges you can get past. There is joy in figuring out how to accomplish challenges, and as you get over the hurdle, they then enhance your life.

Take time to appreciate nature and all the little things that you take for granted when you are outside. Nature brings us a continuing wonder.

A couple of other ways to practice gratitude:

1. I make a list every morning when I get up of 5 things that I am grateful for that happened the day before.
2. Another great time to practice gratitude is at night before you go to sleep. It will calm your busy mind and help you sleep better. Write your gratitude into a journal and then turn off the lights.

3. If you are not a list maker, start a big canning jar and call it your gratitude jar. Deposit a thought of gratitude whenever something happens for which you are grateful.

4. Whenever you have a negative thought, replace it with a positive one. This is called "crowding out," and eventually, you will have more and happier thoughts instead of negative ones.

5. COOK and eat with your family around a dinner table. Make it a family tradition to share what you are grateful for with each other at the family meal. My family also always told funny stories about ourselves from our day. These are precious memories.

6. Make a gratitude collage, similar to a vision board, and include pictures of people in your life that love and support you, your pets, your job if you love it, and what job would if you don't. (See collage at the head of this chapter to see mine.)

7. Volunteer for a local charity and think about how lucky you are. Volunteering also brings "feel good about ourselves" feelings that we can do something great for somebody else.

8. Write and deliver a feel-good letter. It will be something that makes you feel good, and the win is, it makes someone else feel good too.

9. A gratitude practice begins by **paying attention**. Notice all the good things you usually take for granted. Did you sleep well last night? Did someone at work or on the street treat you with courtesy? Have you caught a glimpse of the sky, with its sun and clouds, and had a moment of peace? Did you catch the sunrise and how it danced across the sky? It also involves acknowledging that difficult and painful moments are instructive, and you can be grateful for them as well. I believe there are no victims. Own your life and be grateful for the experiences that you have.

My father would tell me a story, when I was young, that the Easter bunny needed a job when it wasn't Easter, so he painted the sky twice a day. I rarely see a beautiful sunrise or sunset without thinking of my Dad and being grateful that he shared that story with me. It makes me smile.

Part of the point of gratitude is to acknowledge what is good in your life, and it also shows others appreciation.

And it recognizes the good in every aspect of our lives.

Gratitude inspires future hope and lays the groundwork for other wonders to occur.

Gratitude is a relationship-building attitude. Emmons writes, "because it requires us to see how we have been supported by others."

As an employer, gratitude has many benefits.

1. Gratitude recognizes people for their accomplishments.
2. It gives others the incentive(s) to go above and beyond.
3. Gratitude can improve your job performance and give you such a great attitude it helps you to succeed. Gratitude makes you a more effective manager, helps you network, increases your decision-making capabilities, increases your productivity, and helps you get mentors and proteges. As a result, gratitude helps you achieve your career goals, as well as making your workplace a more friendly and enjoyable place to be.
4. Gratitude improves productivity both for you and for your employees because it takes the edge off all those little nagging thoughts and worries.
5. Employees who know they are appreciated have increased productivity. They are happier on the job and work harder.
6. Gratitude increases goal achievement for both you and your team.
7. Gratitude improves your customer service and business growth. Companies you do business with love to be appreciated, and it builds long-lasting bonds.
8. Gratitude results in improved self-esteem.
9. It lets your customers know you are grateful for them, which will help your bottom line.
10. Gratitude to existing customers brings increased referrals for new clients.
11. The Law of Attraction works here. Gratitude, in business, attracts more business.
12. Gratitude cures perfectionism. You start being kinder and gentler with yourself, allowing you to expand and grow.

13. Gratitude allows you to focus on what IS working and then allows the mind to expand upon all your successes.
14. By showing gratitude to your partners, it opens the possibility for greater collaboration and more creativity to occur between you.
15. Gratitude in business allows you to turn challenges into opportunities for growth.
16. Gratitude allows you to focus on what is vital in your business.
17. Gratitude ensures that you take nothing for granted, and that makes you memorable.

What are the benefits of practicing gratitude for your health?

1. If you practice gratitude regularly, it could impact and your lower blood pressure.
2. It multiplies your moments of joy and makes them longer lasting.
3. Once you begin to find things to savor, the feeling is addictive, and you start to look for it everywhere.
4. You will be more likely to exercise.
5. It will reduce feelings of envy and encourages positive emotions.
6. Gratitude boosts your self-esteem. It will increase selflessness and reduce stress.
7. You will be more likely to befriend others who offer support if you express gratitude.
8. It lowers your possibility of coronary artery disease.
9. Gratitude grants us higher levels of alertness, enthusiasm, determination, attentiveness, and energy.
10. It improves sleep duration and quality.
11. It improves immune function.
12. It lowers inflammation.
13. It creates healthier heart rhythms.
14. It reduces stress. "When I am more grateful, I feel more connected with myself and my environment, which reduces stress and brings me happiness."
15. Stress hormones like cortisol are 23% lower in grateful people.

16. Practicing gratitude lengthens telomeres, which are the tips of your DNA, and reduces the effects of aging on the brain.
17. Gratitude floods your brain with feel-good chemicals like serotonin.
18. Gratitude lowers depression.
19. If you practice gratitude, you will have fewer aches and pains and take better care of yourself in general.
20. Gratitude is an effective strategy for reducing insecurity.
21. Gratitude is linked to higher good cholesterol HDL, lower bad cholesterol LDL, and a more positive response to stress.
22. Gratitude creates the possibility of better choices, as to eating healthier and exercising, and the people who practice gratitude are more optimistic.
23. Gratitude improves your relationship with your spouse and your children. No one likes to be taken for granted, and the simple practice of gratitude allows loved ones to feel appreciated.
24. Gratitude doesn't just make you happier; it is happiness in and of itself!

I think we forget to be grateful for the simplest things. But every time we ARE thankful for something, it warms our heart and helps us approach the new day from a positive perspective.

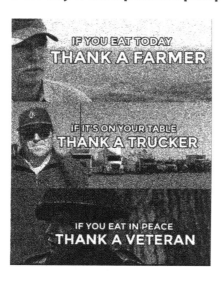

I read an interesting story when I was researching gratitude about a man who was a Larry David type personality that decided to dig down into gratitude. He is described as "a neurotic, obsessive person with a sense of humor" in one of his book reviews. He chose coffee and decided to thank everyone who was involved with his cup of java in the morning. He found over 1000 people to thank for the joy of his cup every morning, and he wrote a book about it called **Thanks a Thousand: A Gratitude Journey**.[76] Simon & Schuster/ TED (November 13, 2018)

His journey took him around the world. He wanted to thank all the people that he had been taking for granted and who enabled him to have his cup of coffee every morning, including farmers, chemists, artists, presidents, truckers, mechanics, biologists, miners, smugglers, and goatherds. Doing this made him happier, more generous, and more connected. He started with the NYC water company and even met a man whose grandfather had been driven from his land to put the water reservoir in. He traveled to Columbia, and the coffee growers were confused that he was grateful for them, because they were so grateful to him for buying and drinking their coffee. He lists the 1000 people he thanked in the back of the book. It certainly makes me stop and think about how many lives were touched by everyday things I take for granted.

In my jewelry years, I had bought a film from the Natural History Museum in Los Angeles that helped me be grateful for all the hands that had touched the gemstones I was making into jewelry. I loaned the film to a customer and never got it back, but it was a fantastic tale of going deep into the mountains of Columbia and how difficult it was to find the gems and then how exciting it was to find them. It was hard work mining for those gems, often with no reward. Once the gem was discovered, getting it out of the mountains to the market was an amazing feat. It then continued its journey by going to a master cutter and then finally got chosen to go into just the right piece of jewelry. It made me stop and contemplate how many hands had touched that gem before it came to market.

We take so much for granted. However, practicing gratitude brings a smile to my heart every morning. I have been blessed with so much and touched by so many people. I am sure I miss some things, but my heart is aware that these people have blessed my life and that my life is better as a result.

One last thought on the subject. I was at a retreat in Sedona last Spring, and I commented in a room full of people that I was very grateful that I got autoimmune disease. People looked at me like I had lost my mind or perhaps that I had landed from Mars. *smile*

I am grateful that I got so sick because my life today is different and happier in so many ways.

- I was in a toxic relationship, and he decided he didn't like that I was sick.
- We broke up, and I went looking for someone to go on a get-well journey with me. I found my current husband and married him five years ago. He is my true soul mate, and he supports me in every way. He wants me to be happy, and he works hard at that every day.
- Both John and I had homes, and they were 10 minutes apart. We sold John's home and purchased a home in Sedona, which to me, is heaven on earth. We have family and friends in LA, so LA will always be our primary residence, so we used the balance of the money from John's home to remodel my home there. I have lived in this home on and off since I was 12. It is full of happy memories, so I am thrilled to be here still.
- I got a new perspective about health, and that I could own my health and find the keys to feeling great again. You don't appreciate your health quite the same way as you do when you no longer have it and regain it. I am grateful that I got the opportunity to turn it around and find my way back.
- I sold my jewelry business to one of my customers. I had been joking before I got sick that I was going to have to hire a helicopter and scatter jewelry over LA to get rid of inventory. I sold the part of my business that was ongoing, and with the balance, I got to contribute tons of jewelry to good causes to help others less fortunate than me. How wonderful was that?
- I found a remarkable Functional MD committed to helping me get well again. I am very grateful for her advice and expertise on how to climb back up to wellness and for her encouragement to ditch the toxins. Her approach is so refreshing, and she is continually approaching my health issues from outside the nine dots. She looks at the entire body and how each thing we do will impact my whole body. She practices root-cause medicine. My hubby is now seeing her as well. I am a HUGE proponent of functional medicine as a result.

- I became a health coach. I am grateful for all the opportunities I have had to give hope to others. I have done well over 100 podcasts as a guest and 15 summits. I have coached several clients back to health and tackled confusing ailments no other person was willing to tackle. I work only with lifestyle changes. I have the community TV show that I am currently filming for my local area. None of this was in my plan until after I got sick. I will be starting my podcast on RHG TV/Voice America mid-2020.
- I have ditched the fear, which was my lifelong nemesis. I am no longer afraid to do anything that I want to do, from writing my first book to going on stage in front of a hundred people. At some point in my life, I figured out the only person who kept me from doing what I wanted to accomplish was ME. That is a gift.
- I no longer have pain. That is huge. Now I want to help others get rid of their pain too!
- I have learned the power of love and gratitude. I have a very good life. I am happy.
- Most importantly, I have learned it's all about how you frame your life experiences. They can stop you in your tracks and make you sad, or they can challenge you to accomplish things you never imagined.

I am grateful that I fell into the second category.

Chapter 14

Beauty is an Inside Job

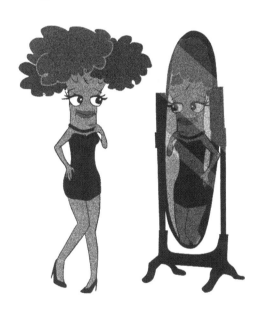

THE BIG TAKEAWAYS ON BEAUTY IS AN INSIDE JOB:[77]

- *Our skin reflects what we are eating, and of how many toxins are in our body.*
- *You are what you eat, and your skin is your showcase to the world.*
- *Toxins can only leave the body in three ways:*
  - *Breathing*
  - *Excretion*
  - *Through your skin.*

Beauty Begins in the Gut

One of my very first clients was a man with annoying psoriasis.

He had tried everything. All the common medications for his issue, every possible lotion and cream, and nothing worked.

I had read that skin issues like psoriasis were a leaky gut issue, and an autoimmune issue, so we set about to see if healing his gut would make a difference. We did what we could to lower his inflammation.

He agreed to change his diet significantly and to eat organic. He limited the amount of sugar he was eating. He took glutathione, and he did stress exercises, and within the first three months saw significant improvements. By lowering his toxic load, his skin got better.

Our skin reflects what we are eating, and of how many toxins are in our body. Clean up now.

You are what you eat, and your skin is your showcase to the world.

Toxins can only leave the body in three ways:

1. Breathing
2. Excretion
3. Through your skin.

The skin is our largest organ. Acne, psoriasis, eczema, even dry skin can all start in the gut.

If you are eating real or fake sugars, GMOs, processed foods, fast food, chemicals sprayed on our crops, chemicals in our water, they go into the gut and need to find a pathway out of the body.

For some people, gluten also creates havoc in the gut and can be reflected in our skin. Some people have sensitivities to other foods, which impact the gut and show up on our skin. I have 15 sensitivities that I now eat around.

There are also unhealthy chemicals in many of our cosmetics. Cosmetics are not regulated, so the toxins that are in them have an easy pathway into the body, and a difficult pathway out.

Even stress and toxic lack of sleep impact the health of the gut, and therefore also the health of our skin.

Have you ever had a hard night's sleep and you look sort of grey in the morning? Poor sleep impacts the skin.

A healthy gut leads to healthy skin and a healthy body. Healing your gut also leads to healthy hair, healthy nails, and a healthy attitude, which are also all part of beauty.

In my book, **It Feels Good to Feel Good, Learn to Eliminate Toxins, Reverse Inflammation, and Feel Great Again**, I discuss how skin conditions such as psoriasis, eczema, and acne are caused by inflammation.

Eczema and psoriasis are autoimmune diseases.

Without getting too technical, autoimmune disease is caused by leaky gut. Food particles are not broken down properly, and then these particles and the toxins get into the bloodstream through a small rip in the gut wall, which is only one cell thick. The rip is caused over time by sugar, alcohol, sensitivities, toxins, gluten, GMOs, infections, parasites, and stress. When the toxins and larger particles of food get through these rips, the rips get larger. Although the gut wall heals itself every seven days, it eventually can't keep up. The body burden is too great. When these particles slip through, the body detects these as foreign substances and screams "attack" because it triggers the immune system. These particles mimic different body systems, wherever the body is weakest, which varies by individual. If it is your skin, it shows up as psoriasis or eczema. On some people, it attacks their thyroid; on other people, it might attack their muscles or their bones. Healing the gut is the first step in reducing the inflammation and in finding relief. Bad skin is one of the early symptoms of leaky gut.

Acne is often a response to conventional dairy. Conventional dairy has lots of cow hormones in it, both natural and synthetic, which then impact the skin. On the other hand, if you are eating grass-fed organic dairy products, they can help with skin issues. Conventional milk is acidic, which can impact your gut.

Acne can also be caused by things put on the skin that block the toxins from coming out. Petroleum jelly products, including mineral oil, can do that. Acne can also be caused by low zinc. It can also be caused by bacteria on the skin, which can be taken care of by dabbing tea tree oil on the skin. (I like the tea tree/lavender blend because it smells better.)

Let's Talk About Unsafe Cosmetic Ingredients

Alcohol, Isopropyl (SD-40): (rubbing alcohol) a very drying and irritating solvent and dehydrator that strips your skin's moisture and natural immune barrier, making you more venerable to bacteria, molds, and viruses. It is made from propylene, a petroleum derivative, and is found in many skin and hair products, fragrance, antibacterial hand washes, as well as shellac and antifreeze. It can act as a "carrier," accelerating the penetration of other harmful chemicals into your skin. It may promote brown spots and premature aging of the skin. A Consumer's Dictionary of Cosmetic Ingredients says it may cause headaches, flushing, dizziness, mental depression, nausea, vomiting, narcosis, anesthesia, and coma. The fatal ingested dose is one ounce or less.

DEA (diethanolamine), MEA (Monoethanolamine) & TEA (triethanolamine): hormone-disrupting chemicals that can form cancer-causing nitrates and nitrosamines. These chemicals are already restricted in Europe due to known carcinogenic effects. In the United States, however, they are still used even though Americans may be exposed to them 10-20 times per day with products such as shampoos, shaving creams, and bubble baths. Dr. Samuel Epstein (Professor of Environmental Health at the University of Illinois) says that repeated skin applications of DEA-based detergents resulted in a major increase in the incidence of liver and kidney cancer. The FDA's John Bailey says this is especially important since "the risk equation changes significantly for children."

DMDM Hydantoin & Urea (Imidazolidinyl): just two of many preservatives that often release formaldehyde, which may cause joint pain, skin reactions, allergies, depression, headaches, chest pains, ear infections, chronic fatigue, dizziness, and loss of sleep. Exposure may also irritate the respiratory system, trigger heart palpitations or asthma, and aggravate coughs and colds. Other possible side effects include weakening the immune system and cancer.

FD&C Color Pigments: synthetic colors made from coal tar, containing heavy metal salts that deposit toxins into the skin, causing skin sensitivity and irritation. Absorption of certain colors can cause depletion of oxygen in the body and death. Animal studies have shown almost all of them to be carcinogenic.

Synthetic Fragrances: mostly synthetic ingredients can indicate the presence of up to four thousand separate ingredients, many toxic or carcinogenic. Symptoms reported to the FDA include headaches, dizziness, allergic rashes, skin discoloration, violent coughing and vomiting, and skin irritation. Clinical observation proves fragrances can affect the central nervous system, causing depression, hyperactivity, irritability, inability to cope, and other behavioral changes.

Alternative—Organic Essential Oils.

Mineral Oil: petroleum by-product that coats the skin like plastic, clogging the pores. Mineral oil interferes with the skin's ability to eliminate toxins, promoting acne, and other disorders. Slows down skin function and cell development, resulting in premature aging. It is used in many products such as baby oil, which is 100% mineral oil!

Alternatives—Moisture Magnets (Saccharide Isomerate) from beets; Ceramides, Jojoba, and other olive oils, etc.

Polyethylene Glycol (PEG): potentially carcinogenic petroleum ingredient that can alter and reduce the skin's natural moisture factor. This could increase the appearance of aging and leave you more vulnerable to bacteria. It is used in cleansers to dissolve oil and grease. It adjusts the melting point and thickens products. (Also used in caustic spray-on oven cleaners.)

Propylene Glycol (PG) and Butylene Glycol: gaseous hydrocarbons which in a liquid state act as "surfactant" (wetting olagents and solvents). They easily penetrate the skin and can weaken protein and cellular structure. They are commonly used to make extracts from herbs. PG is strong enough to remove barnacles from boats! The EPA considers PG so toxic that it requires workers to wear protective gloves, clothing, and goggles and to dispose of any PG solutions by burying them in the ground. Because PG penetrates the skin so quickly, the EPA warns against skin contact to prevent consequences such as brain, liver, and kidney abnormalities. But there isn't even a warning label on products such as stick deodorants, where the concentration is greater than in most industrial applications.

Alternatives—water extracted herbs, Therapeutic Essential Oils, etc.

Sodium Lauryl Sulfate (SLS) & Sodium Laureth Sulfate (SLES): detergents and surfactants that pose serious health threats. Used in car washes, garage floor cleaners, and engine degreasers—and 90% of personal-care products that foam. Beware of these ingredients in shampoos etc. Animals exposed to SLS experienced eye damage, depression, labored breathing, diarrhea, severe skin irritation, and even death. Young eyes may not properly develop if exposed to SLS because proteins are dissolved. SLS may also damage the skin's immune system by causing layers to separate and inflame. When combined with other chemicals, SLS can be transformed into nitrosamines, a potent class of carcinogens. Your body may retain the SLS for up to five days, during which time it may enter and maintain residual levels in the heart, liver, the lungs, and the brain.

Alternative—Ammonium Cocoyl Isethionate.

Triclosan: a synthetic "antibacterial" ingredient—with a chemical structure like Agent Orange! The EPA registers it as a pesticide, giving it high scores as a risk to both human health and the environment. It is classified as a chlorophenol, a class of chemicals suspected of causing cancer in humans. Its manufacturing process may produce dioxin, a powerful hormone-disrupting chemical with toxic effects measured in the parts per trillion; that is only one drop in 300 Olympic-size swimming pools! Hormone disruptors pose enormous long-term chronic health risks by interfering with the way hormones perform, such as changing genetic material, decreasing fertility and sexual function, and fostering congenital disabilities. It can temporarily deactivate sensory nerve endings, so contact with it often causes little or no pain. Internally, it can lead to cold sweats, circulatory collapse, and convulsions. Stored in body fat, it can accumulate to toxic levels, damaging the liver, kidneys, and lungs and can cause paralysis, suppression of immune function, brain hemorrhages, and heart problems. Tufts University School of Medicine says that triclosan is capable of forcing the emergence of "superbugs" that it cannot kill. Its widespread use in popular antibacterial cleaners, toothpaste, and household products may have nightmare implications for our future."

Other Common Toxic Ingredients to Avoid:

- Aluminum
- Phthalates
- DEET
- Dioxins
- Formaldehyde

- PABA
- Para-Aminobenzoic Acid (PABA)
- Parabens
- Phenoxyethanol
- Toluene
- Camphor
- And petroleum jelly products.

Face Powder Can Cause Inhalation Risks

Depending upon the size of the molecules in the powder, if they are small enough, they can cause serious inhalation risks. Talcum powder, mica, Titanium Dioxide, and Zinc Oxide are all used in face powders and can all be small enough to get into areas of the lungs where they cause problems. Talcum powder has additional health hazards. The risks increase if inhaled over several years. This certainly does not support your long-term health.

I offer alternative products in **It Feels Good to Feel Good, Learn to Eliminate Toxins, Reduce Inflammation, and Feel Great Again**. I also explain to you how to research the personal care products that you are currently using and how to research for lower toxin options. Many of the beauty products being purchased are for a visible illusion of beauty, but they do not do anything to enhance your health, which is where the true beauty will come from. The alternative products that I suggest allowing your natural beauty to shine through without the toxins.

The Biggest Key to Healthy Skin and Beauty is in Eating Organic Fruits and Vegetables of All the Colors of the Rainbow

As I discuss in my chapter on how to eat healthily (Chapter 3), I believe in eating real live food that is as close to the farm as possible and in all the colors of the rainbow. You do not need a healthy dose of toxins with your food, so find a way to buy organic. When available, I prefer to eat food that is locally grown. If we would all do that, there would be no need for diet books. Our bodies want to participate in keeping us healthy if we provide the correct building blocks and eliminate all the synthetic chemicals, synthetic ingredients, and fake foods that have penetrated the American diet. The body feels fantastic on real food, and once that is experienced, it becomes a sustainable method of eating and fueling the body. There is no need to "starve" the body short term to lose weight. Eating "healthy and clean" becomes a lifelong strategy.

If you need to lose weight, the internal body needs to be healthy. My favorite book on the subject is Accidentally Overweight by Dr. Libby Weaver. If anything is amuck in your body, it can halt your ability to lose your excess weight. It is NOT about willpower. It is about sugar, fake sugar, hidden MSG, and synthetic ingredients that are hampering your appetite hormones. You need to work on overall health and break your addiction to these substances, and then the weight will automatically start to drop. Throw away your diet books, they don't work and are built on the principles of deprivation, so within a short period, you are back to eating all the foods that created your weight problem from the beginning.

I quoted Deanna Minich, Ph.D., and functional nutritionist in my chapter about the importance of color, and it is worth repeating here.

When it comes to food, crowd out with color rather than restrictive rules. Color is sustainable, creative and engaging, whereas rules are restrictive, demanding, and exhaustive.

DEANNA MINICH, PH.D.—FACEBOOK 10/12/19

If you are struggling with inflammation, it is also impacting how you look. You will be puffy and swollen, and your face will reflect that. It is important to lower your toxic load and to lower your inflammation for your health and for how beautiful you look. Puffy and grey are not a good look.

Cook—It's Crucial for Your Long-Term Health and its Critical for Your Long-Term Beauty.

You control what goes into your body when you cook. It is well worth the effort. By cooking your food and the food for your family, you ensure the quality of nutrients you are putting into your body. And food quality matters.

When cooking at home, you can take any recipe and make it healthy. *There are so many hidden toxins in our food; it is important to cook most of what we are going to eat so that we can control what we are putting into our bodies.*

I avoid using processed foods loaded with chemicals and avoid things like canned soup because of the ingredients and the BPA in the cans.

The body wants to stay healthy. You need to ensure that you are giving it the tools and nutrients to do its job.

The Trouble with Sugar

Sugar impacts our bodies poorly in so many ways. It causes wrinkles; it interferes with important body functions, and it mucks around with the hormones that control hunger. If you are addicted to sugar, you will have no willpower, and continue to eat long after your body is full. It is very important to detox off the sugar to have food freedom and to lose weight. Fake sugars are also poisonous to the body. They are mostly either neurotoxins, or they destroy our gut bacteria. Be careful even of agave, which is very hard on the liver, and most stevia, because of the process used to get the stevia from the leaf. We use powdered green stevia in my house because it is less processed than the stevia in alcohol or white powder.

Sugar in the diet impacts our skin and over time ages it. It's also very hard on our gut.

The Perils of Processed Foods and Synthetic Ingredients

Similarly, to sugar, chemicals in synthetic ingredients in processed and fast foods are created to be addictive and to turn off your hunger hormones. They also are doing the body harm. My rule of thumb is read labels, always, and if you can't pronounce it, or if you don't know what it is, do not buy it and do not eat it. Your body will appreciate this and will help you show up more beautiful to the world.

Why Does Stress Cause Weight Gain?

Stress triggers cortisol, one of our hormones, and puts us into fight or flight mode. This response gives us a burst of energy, changes our metabolism and blood flow, which impacts our digestion and appetite. Cortisol triggers a desire to eat what we know as comfort foods that are generally high in carbohydrates and sugar. Stress impacts us to store belly fat. Using a Belly Button Wand keeps our skin supple and beautiful from the inside out, releasing stress and positively stimulating all our organs.[78]

https://changeyourenergy.com/shop/609/belly-button-healing-kit

How Do Anxious Negative Thoughts Sabotage Our Diet?

One reason you may find yourself binging on carbohydrates when you feel anxious or stressed is that carbohydrates temporarily raise serotonin levels. A powerful neurotransmitter, serotonin affects your emotions, alleviating anxiety, and depression. The temporary lift you get from binging on carbohydrates, though, is often followed by a crash, and it certainly isn't worth the increased calories and resulting weight gain.

What is Functional Medicine?

Functional medicine is a new paradigm in medicine. A functional practitioner has gotten additional training from the Institute for Functional Medicine. My MD graduated from Yale but then got the additional training when she got sick and was looking for a solution. Conventional medicine tends to try to match up the symptoms with a pharmaceutical.

Although a functional MD has the same drugs in her toolbox, her original approach is to find the "root cause" of the ailment. Drugs could be used as a temporary solution. Appointments are longer, and treatments are more inventive. Different tests are taken to identify what is causing the symptom. One major difference is a functional MD reacts before a test shows a disease state and tries to improve the result before the patient enters that disease state.

In my book, It Feels Good to Feel Good, Learn to Eliminate Toxins, Reduce Inflammation, and Feel Great Again, you help people lighten their toxic load and inspire people to eat healthily.

The first part of the book is written to people with chronic pain that don't know where to start to find a solution. The second part of the book identifies where the toxins are—in our food, (which is broken down to organic vs. conventionally grown vs. GMOs, processed foods, canned goods, fast food, dairy, sugar, soda, clean meats, soy, oils), our cosmetics, our over the counter drugs, our kitchens, our cleaning solutions, and our water and then also in our heads—stress, anxiety, lack of sleep, toxic relationships, lack of exercise. I not only identify the toxin, but I also share what I have replaced it with and why, and if you don't like my choice (bio-individuality), I explain how to research to find your own. Once you buy the book, if you write to me, I send you a workbook to use as you read my book. My idea is that since it is all about toxic load, each toxin you eliminate gets you one step closer to health. You write down in the workbook the things that you identify that you want to replace, and then when you run out of the toxic item, you replace it with a much less toxic choice. I wrote the manual that I wish I had had when I got autoimmune disease seven years ago, and I share everything that I have learned. As a result, my book has now won 13 awards.

If you systematically start to lower your toxic load today, you will improve your beauty, and more importantly, you will improve your beauty from the inside out. Remember, **Beauty is an Inside Job**, so treat your body well and eliminate the toxins in your life beginning today.

"If your pretty, you're pretty." But the only way to be beautiful is to be loving. Otherwise, it's just "congratulations about your face."

JOHN MAYER

Finally, my Philosophy About Beauty

Concentrate on being beautiful on the inside, not the outside.

Be:

      Passionate
      Intelligent
      Witty
      Klutzy
      Interesting
      Funny
      Adventurous
      Crazy
      Talented

Be:

      Loving
      Kind
      Compassionate
      Honest
      Ethical
      Present
      Engaged
      Magical
      Live with purpose
      Daring
      Spiritual
      Authentic, always
      Your definition of Amazing

That's what real Beauty is.

And this beauty will touch the hearts and souls of everyone you meet.

It will be a life filled with beauty

And this beauty if far more memorable

It's the Beauty of a Life Well-Lived

For more information on toxins in your personal care products, buy **It Feels Good to Feel Good, Learn to Eliminate Toxins, Reduce Inflammation and Feel Great Again**, available at https://cherylmhealthmuse/book/ or on Amazon.[79]

Chapter 15

Sun Care

**How to protect yourself without the toxins that
are in the majority of SPF products**

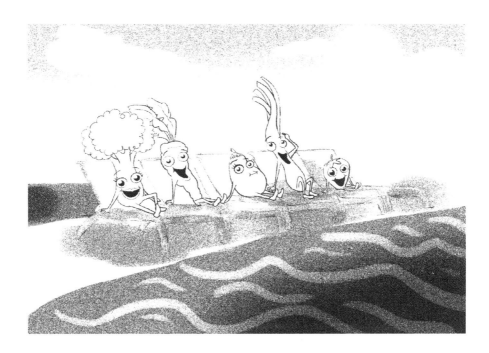

THE BIG TAKEAWAYS ON SUN CARE:[80]

- *The ingredients commonly used in sunscreens have only recently been tested for toxicity.*
- *Sunscreens are designed to stay on the skin for long periods, increasing exposure to what is in them.*
- *Many sunscreen chemicals are absorbed into the body and can be measured in blood, breast milk, and urine samples.*
- *Oxybenzone is an endocrine disrupter.*
- *Avoid all products with added Vitamin A, as it is a suspected carcinogen.*
- *Thank goodness for EWG.org's database, where you can look products up and get the EWG rating from 1-10. (EWG stands for the Environmental Working Group)*
- *High SPF ratings are, according to the FDA, inherently misleading.*

I bet it never occurred to you, but sunscreens are highly toxic. The ingredients commonly used in sunscreens have only recently been tested for toxicity. Sunscreens are designed to stay on the skin for long periods, increasing exposure to what is in them. Many sunscreen chemicals are absorbed into the body and can be measured in blood, breast milk, and urine samples. What they do know is Oxybenzone is an endocrine disrupter. Avoid all products with added Vitamin A, as it is a suspected carcinogen.

Although I hadn't thought about it much in my sunbathing years, I did figure out that some sun products were not my friend. I remember going to the beach with friends when I was in my 30's, and I used one of the most popular suntan gels on my body. It burned so bad; I ran to the showers, which fortunately were close to where we had put down our towels. I got the beginning of blisters on my skin. It was awful. So, discovering that these products were loaded with toxins should not have been a surprise to me, and yet, hark, it was.

Personal care products have not been regulated. The companies themselves are supposed to self-regulate. They use many ingredients that are toxic and harmful to our bodies. Thank goodness for EWG.org's database,[81] where you can look products up and get the EWG rating from 1-10. (EWG stands for the Environmental Working Group) If your specific product is not listed in their database, you can look up the ingredients. Its eye-opening, I must tell you. They also have a guide now for sunscreens and recommendations for safer products.

Check the EWG guide for other safer sunscreens available here.

https://www.ewg.org/sunscreen/

> Note—EWG is a great site to monitor all the toxicity of your products from vegetables, to cosmetics, to the water coming out of your tap. Get familiar with their database.

The FDA is now proposing significant changes in how sunscreen ingredients are evaluated for safety. Several of the commonly used ingredients are endocrine disruptors impacting our estrogen levels and in boys and men, their testosterone levels. Currently, the ingredients have been unregulated, and the FDA is unaware of whether these ingredients cause cancer.

So, what to do instead? We know that prolonged sun exposure also has health implications. Se this is important, but you don't want to use a product that you think is protecting you from the sun but is causing you other health issues.

Follow these recommendations from the Environmental Working Group that studies products, their toxicity, and the implications to our health:

1. Wear clothes and protect your skin from harsh sun exposure.
2. Plan your activities around the sun. Stay in during the hottest and brightest time of the day. Be in the sun in the early morning and late afternoon.
3. Find or create shade. Sit under a tree or put up an umbrella. Keep infants in the shade.
4. If you start to get pink, get out of the sun. Red, blistered, sore skin means you have gotten too many rays. Be aware and be careful.

5. Sunglasses are a must! They aren't worn for fashion; they are protecting your eyes from UV rays.
6. Check the UV index. This will guide you. You can Google it and plan your activities around it.

A couple of other notes:

- High SPF ratings are, according to the FDA, inherently misleading.
- Sunscreens perform imperfect protection.

Some beaches in Hawaii have banned sunscreen products because they were washing off people's skin and killing sea life. Since our skin is our largest organ, think about what these products are doing to YOUR body.

What else can you do?

Find a product that has a low toxin number. I use Keys-Soaps moisturizer under my makeup and on my skin when I am getting sun exposure. This product is rated 2 on a 5-point scale with a range of low to high of 0-5.

https://www.keyspure.com/product-category/skin-antiaging-beauty/sunscreen/

For the rest of my body, I now use Pacifica Sun + Skincare SPF 30 Mineral Sunscreen Coconut Probiotic. It comes in a mini to fit in my pocket, and I used the larger version at home on my way out the door.

Drink lots of filtered water all day long, and it's even more important to stay hydrated when you are out in the sun.

Since you are avoiding the sun, get your Vitamin D levels checked each time you go to the doctor. Your body needs adequate Vitamin D to function properly, and most of us are now deficient. Vitamin D from milk is vitamin D-2 and is synthetic. We need vitamin D-3.

Part VI

Return to Nature

Chapter 16

Indulge in Self-care

It is a necessity of health, and you are worth it

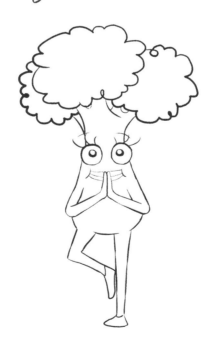

THE BIG TAKEAWAYS ON INDULGE IN SELF CARE:[82]

- *"A car runs out of gas if it's driven without refueling, and it's the same for us; we need to "refuel" with self-care."*

- *Self-care needs to be something you actively plan, rather than something that happens. It is an active choice, and you must treat it as such. Add certain activities to your calendar, announce your plans to others to increase your commitment, and actively look for opportunities to practice self-care.*

- *Create a "no" list, with things you know you don't like, or you no longer want to do. Examples might include: Not checking emails at night, not attending gatherings you don't like, not answering your phone during lunch/dinner.*

- *Promote a nutritious, healthy diet.*

- *Get enough sleep. Adults need 7-8 hours of sleep each night. This is essential to keep your brain healthy.*

- *Exercise. In contrast to what many people think, exercise is as good for our emotional health as it is for our physical health. It increases serotonin levels, leading to improved mood and energy. In line with the self-care conditions, what's important is that you choose a form of exercise that you like! Exercise daily as part of your self-care routine.*

- *Follow-up with medical care. It is not unusual to put off checkups or visits to the doctor.*

- *Use relaxation exercises and/or practice meditation. You can do these exercises at any time of the day.*

- *Spend enough time with your loved ones.*

- *Do at least one relaxing activity every day, whether it's taking a walk or spending 30 minutes unwinding.*

- *Do at least one pleasurable activity every day, from going to the movies, cooking, or meeting with friends.*

- *Look for opportunities to laugh!*

Self-care is the key to living a balanced life.

In my first book, **It Feels Good to Feel Good, Learn to Eliminate Toxins, Reduce Inflammation, and Feel Great Again,** I list 42 different things you can do to practice self-care. I feel so strongly about the importance of self-care I want to revisit the subject in this book and approach it from the point of view of returning to nature. First of all, I want to revisit the basics, and then I want to branch out more deeply on the importance of nature for your physical, emotional, and mental health.

Part of the reason I got autoimmune disease eight years ago was that I wasn't nurturing myself. I was working 24/7 in my business. I was getting up often at 2 AM to catch a flight to the East Coast to meet with customers, and then often returning immediately after the appointment the next day without even giving my body a chance to "catch" my breath. My life was constantly scheduled, not by someone else, but by myself, and taking care of me was not on my program. I missed all the signs that my toxic load was building because I never allowed my mind or my body to be quiet.

"A car runs out of gas if it's driven without refueling, and it's the same for us; we need to "refuel" with self-care."[83]

I wish I had addressed the importance of self-care BEFORE I got sick. But now I do practice it in a variety of ways, and I want to share them with you.

1. Where do you start? Well, there are three golden rules:

    -   Stick to the basics. Over time you will find your rhythm and routine. You will be able to implement more and identify more particular forms of self-care that work for you.
    -   Self-care needs to be something you actively plan, rather than something that happens. It is an active choice, and you must treat it as such. Add certain activities to your calendar, announce your plans to others to increase your commitment, and actively look for opportunities to practice self-care.

- What I often emphasize to my clients is that keeping a conscious mind is what counts. In other words, if you don't see something as self-care or don't do something to take care of yourself, it won't work as such. Be aware of what you do, why you do it, how it feels, and what the outcomes are.

Although self-care means different things to different people, there's a basic checklist that can be followed by all of us:

- Create a "no" list, with things you know you don't like, or you no longer want to do. Examples might include: Not checking emails at night, not attending gatherings you don't like, not answering your phone during lunch/dinner. Leaning to say no to you is also important, no to more sugar, no to spending silly money that will impact your budget, etc.
- Promote a nutritious, healthy diet.
- Get enough sleep. Adults need 7-8 hours of sleep each night. This is essential to keep your brain and your body healthy.
- Exercise. In contrast to what many people think, exercise is as good for our emotional health as it is for our physical health. It increases serotonin levels, leading to improved mood and energy. In line with the self-care conditions, what's important is that you choose a form of exercise that you like! **Exercise daily as part of your self-care routine.**
- Follow-up with medical care. It is not unusual to put off checkups or visits to the doctor.
- Use relaxation exercises and/or practice meditation. You can do these exercises at any time of the day. (See Chapter 12 on stress.)
- Spend enough time with your loved ones.
- Do at least one relaxing activity every day, whether it's taking a walk or spending 30 minutes unwinding.
- Do at least one pleasurable activity every day, from going to the movies, cooking, or meeting with friends.
- Look for opportunities to laugh!
- Practice gratitude.

2. Take care of yourself by taking care of your gut.
3. Food Quality Matters. Eat organic and avoid GMOs to keep your body vibrant. Enjoy all the colors of the rainbow.
4. Take a self-care trip. Go on a retreat. Refresh yourself and rejuvenate.
5. Go to a day spa with a girlfriend and spoil yourself.
6. Get his and hers massages with your sweetheart. John and I spoil each other regularly.
7. Take a self-care break by getting outside. Walk around the block. Use all your senses. Listen to the sounds, see the sky and the birds and the trees, feel the bark of a tree, or put your hands into the dirt, smell some flowers. Grow herbs and take them inside and "taste" them.
8. Let a pet help you with your self-care.

None of these things take up so much time that they interrupt your workday or what you can accomplish. All of them increase your productivity. My next two chapters are a deep dive into other things I have learned for self-care. All of this is important, and you are worth it!

Chapter 17

New Thoughts on Self-Care - The Importance of Alone Time

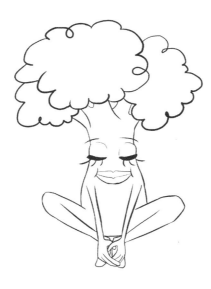

THE BIG TAKEAWAYS ON THE IMPORTANCE OF ALONE TIME:[84]

- *If you don't take care of yourself, you don't have anything left to keep taking care of everyone else.*

- *I am a very social person, but sometimes I come to a place where I am "over-peopled."*

- *Mix your alone time with productivity, relaxation, and meditation or self-reflection.*

- *The more time you spend with yourself and fill your time with intentional productivity, self-care, and love, solitude will change from a generally lonely feeling into a positive time of growth in your life.*

- *Go out into nature and enjoy the outdoors.*

- *Breathe.*

- *Ask your body, "how do you feel?" and then be quiet and let your body answer.*

When I wrote my first book, I shared many ideas that were relatively commonplace for self-care and highlighted the ones that I was regularly doing. Altogether, I noted 42 different ways to take care of you. If you don't take care of yourself, you don't have anything left to keep taking care of everyone else.

In this chapter, I want to talk about nourishing yourself through alone time. I also want to talk about the importance of getting outdoors for self-care, and how important it is to return to nature as often as possible Then, I have a chapter on Forest Bathing and all of the rather incredible reasons why this is so good for your body and soul.

These chapters are a deeper dive into taking care of yourself.

So, let's start with the importance of finding some alone time, which I think is at the core of taking care of you.

I am a very social person, but sometimes I come to a place where I am "over-peopled." When I reach that point, I must get some alone time, or I am not present for the people that I love.

Foster Weekly Alone time as part of your self-care.

It is so important to spend time daily in silence. When I first get up in the morning, I have a morning routine before I even get out of bed where I stretch and twist, and if I can, I go where I can observe the sunrise. In Sedona, one of my great joys is watching the sunrise over the high bluff that I can see out of my kitchen window and appreciate all the beauty that I can enjoy by being in Sedona. This time is my alone time. When I sit down at my desk, the first thing I do every morning is to write down five things I am grateful for at that very moment in time. Even if my hubby gets up as early as I do, he now has adjusted that he should not come and chat with me this early. I tease him that when he gets up, he is like a Chatty Cathy doll[85], and as much as I love him, it rattles me. So, he now politely waits until he hears movement from my office to come and give me my morning kiss and start our day together.

Mix your alone time with productivity, relaxation, meditation or self-reflection.

The more time you spend with yourself and fill your time with intentional productivity[86], self-care, and love, solitude will change from a generally lonely feeling into a positive time of growth in your life. Foster your "alone time." Once you go through the window of lonely to aloneness, you will savor your alone time. You will not be lonely again. I revel in my alone time.

I am starting a new habit of keeping a victory journal. Each morning when I get up, I write down my victories from the day before. This was an idea from my book coach, Lea Woodford that came up in a meeting with my coauthors in her book group. I actually published my victory and gratitude journal, so it is also available for you to use. It is available on Amazon and it is available on my publishing site Heavenly Tree Press.

As women, we don't give ourselves credit for all the amazing things that we accomplish daily, weekly, and monthly. I am almost oblivious to my many achievements. When I stop and think of everything, I have accomplished in the eight years since I got sick, sometimes I am blown away, and yet, if someone asks me what my recent victories are, I have to stop and think. Even worse, I might tell you what I haven't accomplished yet.

Keeping a victory journal[87] will be my way of celebrating me and staying present with where I am and where I want to go.

How to Practice Aloneness:

1. The most important step is to not react to the impulse to reach out to someone to fill your time and space. This is key!
2. Make sure that your loved ones honor your space in your special times you have set to be alone.
3. Try Journaling what is on your mind. Often our heads are so full of thoughts and information, find a way to write them down, and let them go. It allows me to start the day on a new page.
4. In Sedona, there are very powerful vortexes. Some are female, where the energy flows in a counterclockwise direction, whereas others are male, where the energy flows in a clockwise direction. It is believed that when you are in a female vortex, you need to say thank you and release the past for lessons learned. When you are in a male vortex energy, you can manifest the future. What fascinates me is that the tree trunks twist in the direction of the energy of the vortex. Practicing these two disciplines is an important element of alone time for me.
5. Whether or not you have the advantage of using the vortexes, it is always good to practice being grateful for what has come before and to make plans to manifest where you want to go. These are great subjects for your journaling.
6. Go out into nature and enjoy the outdoors. If you live in an urban area, you can still walk and take in your surroundings. Find a local park to walk in. Use all your senses to enjoy your environment. If you decide to walk with a partner, make an agreement to walk together but not to

communicate for a certain part of your walk so that you can "feel" and enjoy the outdoors.

7. Breathe. We need to pay more attention to taking deep breaths. Practice breathing in your alone time. Slow your breathing down and take deeper breaths. Breathe from your lower gut for a while, then breath from your lungs. Breathe from your heart. Make your breathing slow and measured. This will relax your body and put you into a more mindful state.

8. Ask your body, "how do you feel?" and then be quiet and let your body answer. I honestly missed all the signs that my body was showing me that my toxic load was building. I now touch in with my body daily. Your body wants to heal you. And it will let you know if you are doing the things that are making it run optimally or not. You must get quiet and "listen" to it. Your alone time is an excellent time to do this.

9. Find something to do each day that is creative. This will mean different things for different people. For me, it could be developing more art characters to visually encourage others to be healthy (my jubilant broccoli and my triumphant carrot.) Or, for me, it might be cooking a healthy creative dinner. For you, it will be other things. Just set aside time where your creativity can come out to play.

10. Be mindful in your aloneness and stay in the now. Change your thoughts. Change your life. Change the world.

11. You can feel the benefits of aloneness and mindfulness in as little as 15 minutes. Nature restores us mentally and emotionally the same way food and water restore our bodies. Enjoy it often.

Chapter 18

Experience the outdoors and enjoy nature for your health

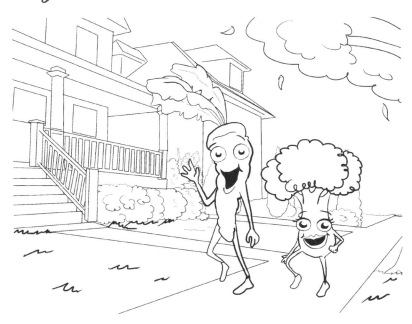

THE BIG TAKEAWAYS ON GETTING OUTDOORS:[88]

> - *Getting outdoors can be taking a walk in your neighborhood, going to a city park to walk, heading to the beach to sit on the sand or at the end of a wharf to watch the waves, or heading to the woods to enjoy forest bathing.*
> - *There are so many benefits to getting off your duff and heading outdoors.*
> - *There are many benefits of being outside in the sunlight. Some of those benefits are:*
>   - *Improved attention spans (short-term and long-term).*
>   - *Increased levels of serotonin (the feel-good neurotransmitter).*
>   - *Increased brain activity in those areas responsible for empathy and emotional stability.*
>   - *Increased energy levels, from just 20 minutes outside per day.*

Getting outdoors can be taking a walk in your neighborhood, going to a city park to walk, heading to the beach to sit on the sand or at the end of a wharf to watch the waves, or heading to the woods to enjoy forest bathing. I wrote an entire chapter (19) on forest bathing. In this chapter, I want to discuss the other two options, getting outdoors as an urbanite, and getting outdoors to return to a more natural setting.

There are so many benefits to getting off your duff and heading outdoors.

1. Being outdoors clears your head and soul.
2. Going outdoors allows you to soak in Vitamin D, which is critical for your body to function. Most of us are now deficient in Vitamin D. You cannot get it from dairy, which is synthetic Vitamin D-2. You need it from the sun as vitamin D-3 or from a quality supplement. Enjoy it from the sun as often as you can.
3. Grab whatever little bit of nature and the outdoors you can get now. It could be in the wild, it could be in a park, it could be taking a walk in your neighborhood, it could be relaxing in your back yard, or it could be as

simple as looking out your window at a beautiful day. Any of these will reduce your stress and give you an important mental break.

4. You can leave any anxiety or worry at the door by leaving your routine. Spend time healing by experiencing the out of doors.

5. You can empty your mind by returning to nature, which is when I am my most creative. Random thoughts pop into my mind when I am outside, and if I get quiet and catch these thoughts, they often can grow into great ideas.

6. Whatever problems you leave behind when you enter the outdoors can create a new perspective. Your problems become smaller. You can relax with them.

7. There are many places outdoors to find calm. For me, it has always been water. I used to mentally throw my problems into the ocean by going out on one of the many wharves at the beach in Southern California. I love the many moods of the ocean. Lately, my place to soothe my soul is among the trees, or in the red rocks of Sedona, my second home. I love to sit along the Verde River in Sedona and let the water of the river soothe me as I sit in the trees at the water's edge.

8. If possible, we need to feel the joy of the sun on our skin. It warms us and brings us happiness. In the winter, in some areas of the country where it gets dark in the winter, there is something called Seasonal Affective Disorder, so on sunny days, it is imperative to get out of doors to revel in the glory of sunlight. Without the sun, we experience vitamin deficiency and can experience mental depression.

9. Numerous studies have been conducted to establish the benefits of spending time in nature; some of those benefits are:[89]
   - Improved attention spans (short-term and long-term).
   - Increased levels of serotonin (the feel-good neurotransmitter).
   - Increased brain activity in those areas responsible for empathy and emotional stability; and
   - increased energy levels, from just 20 minutes outside per day.

10. Get outside and practice grounding. Go barefoot in the grass (that hasn't been sprayed with Roundup). Draw the electrical charges into your body and let them flow through you. I am lucky in Sedona because I

can go and enjoy one of the many vortexes in the area. There are many health benefits to doing this: better sleep, better immunity, and a better connection to the Earth. It is still important when I am in suburbia in Los Angeles to get outside and put my feet in the grass and to ground.

11. You will be happier after getting outdoors.

12. True health comes from doing the things that encourage our wellbeing. Getting outdoors is certainly one of the most important things we can do for ourselves.

13. Being outdoors allows you to work on your spiritual health. Open your senses to the wonders of our world and practice gratitude that we have these many wonders to enjoy. Bathe in whatever greater power you believe in.

14. Mother Nature's love for us is unconditional. When we need shelter from the heat, we can retreat to the shade of beautiful trees. When we need warmth, we can bask in the sun. When we need darkness so that we can sleep, the sun retreats and creates nightfall.[90] Nature is a miracle and complex, and loving and sometimes challenging, but she regenerates. I once commented to my husband that we humans are killing the Earth. He replied that the Earth would survive, but we may not survive as a species on the Earth. ***We need to protect it and do what we can to save ourselves***. It is important for our wellbeing that we stop making the Earth sick. Being in nature gives us a new attitude to what she offers our lives.

15. Eat in a way that connects you to nature. Real food heals. Eat foods from a farm as close to you as possible so that you get maximum nutrition from the plant. Eat in season. Enjoy all the colors of the rainbow. Don't eat chemicals on or in your food.

16. If possible, garden. Get your fingers in the dirt. It could be herb pots on your kitchen windowsill or pots with veggies and tomatoes on your porch. Or, it could be a plot in your back yard where you grow seasonal veggies.

"We don't have to heal the Earth; she can heal herself. All we have to do is stop making her sick. To this simple truth, I would add that she can heal us as well."

LAKOTA SHAMAN WALLACE BLACK ELK

Chapter 19

Back to Nature and the Benefits of Forest Bathing

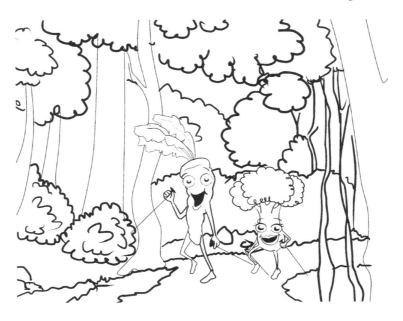

THE BIG TAKEAWAYS ON RETURNING TO NATURE AND THE BENEFIT OF FOREST BATHING:[91]

- *Forest Bathing comes to us from Japan, where many studies have been conducted about the benefits of going deep into the forest.*

- *Forest bathing or spending time in nature has become a cornerstone of preventive health care and healing in Japanese medicine. It is part of Dao philosophy and other Eastern approaches to health.*

- *There are many psychological and physical health benefits of forest bathing.*

- *Research also shows that "forest bathing positively creates calming neuro-psychological effects through changes in the nervous system, reducing the stress hormone cortisol and boosting the immune system."*

- *"Trees shower (or bathe) themselves in an antimicrobial, antifungal, antibacterial compound called phytoncides," explains Ben Page, founder of Shinrin Yoku LA. "This is how trees combat disease."*

- *When people breathe in these chemicals, our bodies respond by increasing the number and activity of a type of white blood cell called natural killer cells or NK. These work to thwart cancer.*

- *One day in the forest enhances our natural killer cells for up to seven days. In two or three days, the effects can last for 30 days.*

- *Chemicals called "terpenes." are released by some plants. Terpenes come from leaves, pine needles, tree trunks, and thick bark. They also are released from bushes, herbs, shrubs, mushrooms, mosses, and ferns. They enter our bodies through our skin and our lungs. Terpenes are anti-inflammatory, anti-tumorigenic, and neuroprotective. Terpenes are also anti-cancer chemicals.*

- *Forest bathing is about "non-doing" and practicing the art of being.*

"Thousands of tired, nerve-shaken, over-civ-ilized people are beginning to find out that going to the mountains is going home.

Wilderness is a necessity."

JOHN MUIR 1838-1914

"Forest therapy was founded on the idea that as a species, we spent the first few million years of our existence in the forest. Now we reside in cities and suburbs and are surrounded by all kinds of stimuli. This has led to stress that results in negative health consequences.[92]"

The John Muir quote above is over 100 years old and yet is truer today than perhaps even when he first wrote the words.

Research has shown that even 5 minutes in nature can lower blood pressure, relax muscles, and increase connection with others.

So let's talk about forest bathing and spending time in nature and its importance to the human body and the human mind.

Forest bathing is a literal translation of *shinrin-yoku*, a term coined by the Japanese government in 1982 to encourage urbanites to immerse themselves in nature.[93] The Japanese take this so seriously that they certify their best forests for bathing.

Forest bathing or spending time in nature has become a cornerstone of preventive health care and healing in Japanese medicine. It is part of Dao philosophy and other Eastern approaches to health.

Especially in this age where so many of us are urbanites, it is increasingly important that we spend time outdoors and in nature.

I will admit, I don't always take advantage of forest bathing or being out of doors when I am in Los Angeles, even though I live at the base of 5000 ft mountains with lots of forests. However, it is an important reason that I love living part-time in Sedona. Just being in my back yard brings serenity as well as the ability to walk along the Verde river and sit in the trees or to be out of doors in the tremendous beauty of the area.

"The idea is simple: if a person simply visits a natural area and walks in a relaxed way, there are calming, rejuvenating, and restorative benefits.[94]"

We know this intuitively, but we often do not make time in our busy lives to enjoy a consistent practice.

Forest bathing includes walking outdoors in parks and urban areas. You don't need to drive a hundred miles to enjoy the activity and the benefits of forest bathing. Find a local place to walk and enjoy the outdoors.

"Biophilia "is a term made famous by entomologist E.O. Wilson. "It means humans are hard-wired to connect with nature."

In May 2019, Aaron Ruben of Outdoor Magazine reported that the growing research on the mental health impacts of access to green spaces means that more and more doctors are prescribing time in nature to patients.[95]

The benefits of "forest bathing" include:[96]

- Boosted immune system
- Reduced blood pressure
- Reduced stress
- Improved mood
- Reduced anger
- Reduced anxiety
- Helps fight cancer cells[97]
- Increased ability to focus, even in children with ADHD
- Accelerated recovery from surgery or illness
- Increased energy level
- Improved sleep

- Deeper and clearer intuition
- Increased flow of energy
- Increased capacity to communicate with the land and its species
- Increased flow of eros/life force
- Deeper friendships
- Increased happiness
- Improved mood, and an excellent antidote for depression
- Reduced cortisol, your stress hormone.
- Can protect against Type II Diabetes[98]
- Improved self-esteem and confidence
- increased passion for life[99]
- Improved connection to life energy[100]

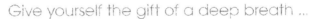

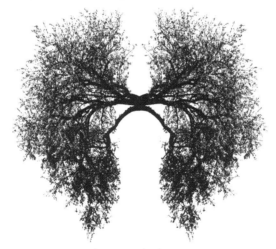

deannaminch.com

I want to point a couple of these out.

- Better sleep—a new study at UC Berkeley concludes that 7 hours of quality sleep is even more important for health than reducing stress.

Being outdoors, and away from artificial lights, helps synchronize your biology to natural circadian rhythms.[101] Research shows that 21[102] different varieties of trees breath and they have a circadian rhythm. They sleep at night. Their tree limbs lower at night. This impacts our circadian rhythms.[103]

- Stress reduction-Chronic stress impacts every organ in your body. It is a key element of "leaky gut," which is at the root of chronic illness.
- Reduced blood pressure -- blood pressure significantly impacts the heart and reduces the likely hood of heart disease.
- Improved mood—most people that I talk to think depression is something they inherited. They do not realize that most serotonin is produced in the gut. This is one of the first things I suggest if someone is depressed. I also suggest that they eat more vegetables in all the colors of the rainbow to return balance to their body and to help manufacture more "feel-good" hormones. I know that if I am feeling down, I can often connect it to what I have been eating, and by correcting to eating more vegetables, my mood will lighten.

The simple concept of stopping to smell the flowers is now proven to improve mood and well-being. "Chinese Medicine Practitioners believe flowers help us manage our emotions and cultivate desired qualities like joy or peace. Their vibrant colors stimulate our senses, triggering the production of melatonin, a calming hormone, and serotonin, a hormone that elevates our mood. Bonus, spending time outdoors among flowers, invites "magical" beings like butterflies, hummingbirds, and dragonflies, inspiring a sense of wonder and awe, which puts minor stressors, like traffic, into perspective."[104]

Research also shows that "forest bathing positively creates calming neuro-psychological effects through changes in the nervous system, reducing the stress hormone cortisol and boosting the immune system."[105] In only 15 minutes of forest bathing blood pressure drops, stress levels are lower, and concentration and mental clarity improve.[106]

"The researchers were able to demonstrate that, compared to a typical city environment, profound health benefits were observed in the subjects when they experienced *Shinrin-yoku*. Across the board, all the measured parameters were significantly better when subjects were in nature, including lower blood pressure, pulse rate, salivary cortisol level, and better heart rate variability."[107]

"Trees shower (or bathe) themselves in an antimicrobial, antifungal, antibacterial compound called phytoncides," explains Ben Page, founder of Shinrin Yoku LA. "This is how trees combat disease."[108] These chemicals also have positive impacts on the human body. These chemicals help the human body fight cancer cells."[109]

When people breathe in these chemicals, our bodies respond by increasing the number and activity of a type of white blood cell called natural killer cells or NK. Forest bathing also encourages "natural killer cells" that protect the human body. These work to thwart cancer.[110] One day in the forest enhances our natural killer cells for up to 7 days.[111] In two or three days, the effects can last for 30 days.[112]

Chemicals called "terpenes." are released by some plants. Terpenes come from leaves, pine needles, tree trunks, and thick bark. They also are released from bushes, herbs, shrubs, mushrooms, mosses, and ferns. They enter our bodies through our skin and our lungs. Terpenes are anti-inflammatory, anti-tumorigenic, and neuroprotective. Terpenes are also anti-cancer chemicals.[113]

These chemicals vary by the season, which makes sense. Terpenes are highest in the summer and lowest in the winter.

*"The clearest way into the Universe
is through a forest wilderness."*

JOHN MUIR

Make going into nature for a half an hour a priority of your week.

- Go to clear your busy mind.
- Leave your goals and expectations behind you as you step onto your path for your walk.
- Leave your phone electronics behind. These have no use as you "bathe" and will interrupt your experience.

- Breathe
- Be present in the experience
- Use all your senses to enjoy the walk.
- Practice a sound-bathing exercise, where all your attention is on the sounds of the area you are in, be it in a forest or an urban park. Let the sounds flow over and through you.
- Use all your senses as you "forest bathe." Hear the sounds, smell the natural scents, see the beauty all around you, touch the different textures, sense the feeling of hot and cold on your skin, (the coolness of the air in the shade, the warmth of the sun on your skin.) Breathe in the clean air.
- Enjoy the walk. Stop to enjoy the beauty of the area that you have chosen. Meander rather than walk fast, and "smell the roses."
- If you go with friends, agree to be silent until the end of your walk.
- I recommend that you stand by a tree and concentrate on breathing with it. You give it your carbon dioxide. The tree gives you its oxygen. I once mentally communicated with a tree, and it was a beautiful experience. Clear your mind and see if you can receive communication from a tree. Pick one of the large matriarchs in the forest to practice.
- Don't stay in the perimeter. The health benefitting chemicals are dense, where the forest is dense. Go into the forest and then relax and "bath" in these amazing chemicals."[114]
- If it has rained, these chemicals are even stronger with greater benefits.
- Stop and enjoy the simplicity of little things, the beauty of a leaf, a sensational wildflower, the height of the Mother tree of the area. Smell the air and enjoy the fragrance.
- Find a place to sit and take in the experience. Notice how the animals and birds adjust to your presence. Listen to the sounds and let them soothe you.
- Feel the dirt beneath your feet and ground to the earth.
- Try a rainbow walk where you look out for objects that are red, orange, yellow, green, blue, and purple. Take pictures of examples of each color that you find in your forest.

Forest bathing is about non-doing and practicing the art of being.[115]

Take long breaths deep into the abdomen. Extending the exhalation of air to twice the length of the inhalation sends a message to the body that it can relax and allows you to enjoy the experience completely.

Forest bathing can be a shared or group activity.

Forest bathing can be guided or independent,

Forest bathing can spark creativity and or problem-solving.

Forest bathing promotes wellbeing.

And don't forget the impact of having live plants in your office and living space. There are benefits just from being surrounded by plants.

Part VII

Poisons in the Home

Chapter 20

How to Get Rid of Bugs Without "...cides" or Poison

THE BIG TAKEAWAYS ON HOW TO GET RID OF BUGS WITHOUT "...CIDES" OR POISON:[116]

- *Avoid pesticide sprays to eliminate insects. Products ending in "...cides" mean that they kill. They are toxic and can cause you harm.*

- *I was fortunate to meet Richard Bugman Fagerland, who has 50 years of experience removing bugs in a non-toxic way. He gave me permission to share his solutions with you.*

How you deal with bugs is important. As we discussed when I was talking about pesticides and herbicides, the suffix "...cides" means kills something. That also means, in most instances, that the substance with the "...cide" on the end of the word is toxic and can harm. It could harm you, your children, and your pets.

I never liked products like Raid. I knew that the stuff that came out of the can was not good for my kitties or me. It was loaded with toxins, and it would get into my nose and lungs and, therefore, into my body. It was also entering my body through my skin.

I hired a caretaker for my mother some years ago who would go berserk with the Raid can whenever she saw ants or bugs. I didn't want these chemicals around my Mom, who had a rare disease. I had to find alternative solutions because I didn't want the stuff in my house or around my cats, long before I got an autoimmune disease, so I have been using these solutions now, in some cases, for many years.

I was lucky to be introduced to Richard Bugman Fagerland recently. He has been an insect expert for more than 50 years. He sold me his books about safe solutions for insects and gave me permission to use his materials freely. I have endnotes on his comments. He, too, is committed to no "…cides," and his experience is invaluable to take care of any insect issue you may have.

Mosquitoes

I have always been a beacon to attract any bug in a 10-mile radius, and this is especially true for mosquitos. Just kidding, but seriously, they find me and dive-bomb me. I have always been particularly yummy to mosquitos, and for the life of me, I do not know why. My husband likes to tease me that it's because I am so sweet. Ha!

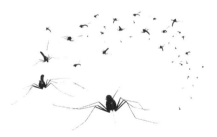

Generally, mosquito activity begins when the temperature warms up to the 50°F level, and mosquitos breed in stagnant water. This can include:[117]

- Flowerpots
- Ponds, marshes, and bogs
- Birdbaths
- Puddles

- Rainwater barrels
- Empty tires or debris in the yard can fill up with water during a rain
- Ditches
- Untended yards
- Heavy shaded areas and long grasses

I don't have any stagnant water.

If I go into my backyard at dinner time to pick lemons, I know that I am going to be instantly attacked. I have a solution which I will share further into the chapter, but if I don't take the time, to do it, I pay dearly.

Before I started to write this chapter, I looked up what it is that attracts mosquitos, and in general, it should not be me. But ever since I was little, I seem to attract them more than the other people around me, so I have found solutions that work for me that I want to share with you.

Let's start with WHY experts think some mosquitos zoom in on some people and not on others.[118]

1 **Apparel**—Mosquitos have good eyesight and head directly for people in dark clothing. Ok, that would be me. I wear a lot of black. But I didn't as a kid, so who can figure?

2 **Blood type**—This is fascinating because mosquitos like people with O blood type. That would be my husband. But they don't like him, they come directly for me, and I am an A. They aren't supposed to like the taste of my blood at all, and B blood types are in the middle.

3 **Gas**—Mosquitos like big people. Ok, I am not a small person, and supposedly I exhale more because of my size. This certainly, wasn't true when I was a kid. And mosquitos like our heads, which is why they buzz around our ears, one of the most annoying things about them. They love carbon dioxide. Ducky.

4 **Heat and sweat**—Mosquitoes have a nose for other scents besides carbon dioxide; they can sniff down victims through the lactic acid, uric acid, ammonia, and other compounds emitted in sweat. This one is weird

because one of my problems is that I have MTHFR, which means what goes into my body stays in my body. I do not detox easily, and I do not sweat. So, why me? As a result of not sweating, I do run warmer than most people, which puts me back in their sights. But I don't do strenuous exercise, which would be a bonus for them. Again, it makes no sense. Nevertheless, they find me easily.

5   **Lively skin**—This one is also interesting. Mosquitos are attracted to people who have more bacteria on their skin. What? I shower daily. But apparently, I emit a lovely fragrance of bacteria. I have the microbes that mosquitos love. This is the explanation for why mosquitos are drawn to ankles and feet, which is certainly true for me, and these areas are a ripe source for bacteria.

6   **Pregnancy**—Mosquitos find pregnant women especially delicious. Again, that would not be me. As you know, I am 71. What you don't know about me is that my biggest regret is that I never had children. The tummies of pregnant women are hotter than the tummies of non-pregnant women. Lucky them.

7   **Time of day**—Some mosquitos are active during the day. Others are most active at night, dusk, or dawn. For most species of mosquito in the United States, their activity peaks during the dusk hours.

8   **Beer**—And finally, apparently, mosquitos like women who drink beer. Maybe if the women are slightly drunk, they are easier to catch? Again, that's not me. I have had fewer beers than the fingers on one hand in my entire life. I don't care for the taste, but that hasn't stopped mosquitos from loving the taste of me.

I have several suggestions as to what to do to protect you from these annoying insects.

My first suggestion is for Tea Tree Oil, and it comes with a story.

Before I write anything, never put any essential oil directly onto your skin. They are strong and could be irritating to your skin. I usually dilute essential oils with coconut oil, making a paste. You will see what I recommend down below. Try it on a small section of your skin first, and if you do not react hostilely, go on to follow my instructions. Make sure you are using real oils, not synthetic oils. I do not use DoTerra or Young Living; I use Rocky Mountain. I have never been a multi-level marketing person. Why should 20+ people make money from my purchase? I love the quality that I get from Rocky Mountain, and the money exchange is just between them and me.

Now, on with my story.

I was in Asia, with my female business partner at the time, Jill[119], and we were in the VIP room at the Calcutta airport. I think we were sitting in the oldest upholstered chairs ever made. They were worn and frayed, but comfortable. Suddenly, I got a big bite. Something that was in or on the chair had bitten me. Probably not a mosquito, but something that bit and made big itchy bumps.

I had tea tree oil with me, so I went to the women's room, wet my hanky, put tea tree oil on it, added more water, and rubbed it everywhere that skin was showing. I returned to my chair and offered my hanky to my partner.

She said ugh, that stuff stinks (and I will admit it's not the nicest smell), but I thought she should use it anyway. She refused. By the time we landed in Bangkok, I still had only the one bite, and Jill was covered from head to toe with large welts. We checked into the hotel and then got the hotel car directly to the emergency room. She lived, but she had big itchy welts, and I was grateful that I had used the tea tree oil.

I have used tea tree oil ever since to protect myself from bugs when I go outside. I use a washcloth, wet it, add tea tree essential oil to it, wet it again, and then rub it all over my skin. Then I go outside to pick my lemons. It works for me. The mosquitos leave me alone. If I don't use it, I get tons of welts. It's as if, when I walk out the back door, I ring the bell and call "dinners on" to all mosquitos in my backyard if I don't use my oils.

When I first met my hubby, he was scheduled on an around the world cruise. I gave him a bottle of the tea tree oil as a bon voyage present. He came back believing it was a lifesaver. Everyone else was getting eaten alive, and he got no bites.

Caution

Tea Tree Oil is unhealthy and toxic for both cats and dogs. If you use it, and you have fur babies, wash your hands and skin well when you return to your home.

Now in researching for this chapter, I have learned that there isn't enough evidence that Tea Tree Oil works. (They didn't ask me. Ha!) I did switch some years ago to a tea tree/lavender combo essential oil, and lavender is listed as a better choice. I switched because it smells better.

But I share with you that it works well for me.

I had learned three years ago. That I needed to keep tea tree oil away from my kitties, they would get one whiff, and they would be gone. I didn't realize that essential oils can be hard on animals and can even poison them, and tea tree oil is one of them. Lavender is also toxic to cats, but not to dogs.

If you are using any essential oils around your pets, be very aware of the animal's reaction to the essential oil.

I have one other suggestion that works for me like a charm. I buy insect spray from Keys Pure. I love all the Keys products. Their insecticide is a one on a 10-point scale for toxicity. (Which means low toxin.) The great thing about their bug spray is that usually, you get a bite before you react, and this spray soothes the bite and then repels the bugs. Again, I spray it on my fingers and then apply it to my skin. https://www.keyspure.com/product/forcex/ This does have some peppermint in it, but my cats never reacted hostilely to it. Peppermint is another oil to keep away from cats.

Keys-pure line product that soothes bug bites is their Broad-Spectrum Insect Repellent Spray

- Repels 200+ Flying & Crawling Insects
- Anti-Parasitic
- Migrating Fast Coverage
- Antiseptic
- Anti-Fungal
- Anti-Itch

They combine high concentrations of Neem oil and Karanja oil with peppermint, red thyme, and lemongrass oil to create a dog-friendly insect repellent.

Again, caution for cat owners. Peppermint is toxic to cats as well.

I just bought the definitive guide to essential oils and their uses. **Essential Oil Safety: A Guide for Health Care Professionals** by Robert Tisserand (Author), Rodney Young Churchill Livingstone; 2 edition (November 6, 2013) My kitties all passed last year, but I want to know more because the last thing I ever want to do is hurt a fur baby.

So, what does EWG recommend? The Environmental Working Group has some surprising recommendations.

"DEET is a reasonable choice when used as directed, even for children. Still, after reviewing the evidence, EWG researchers concluded that it is best to use the lowest effective concentration of DEET, even though it's effective and generally safer than is commonly assumed." DEET is a neurotoxin, so this surprised me, but I trust EWG so you might consider this.

EWG's second recommendation is Picaridin as an alternative to DEET. "It effectively repels both mosquitoes and ticks and, compared to other repellents, is less likely to irritate eyes and skin" What is Picaridin? It's related to Black Pepper. "The EPA says that picaridin has not induced developmental problems in the offspring of animals exposed to it—the chemical harmed young animals only when their mothers had been exposed to doses so high, they were toxic."[120]

"EWG research indicates that, in general, "natural" bug repellent ingredients like castor, cedar, citronella, clove, geraniol, lemongrass, peppermint, rosemary and/or soybean oils are often not the best choice."

For a short duration, EWG recommends a solution of 10% for either Picaridin or DEET. For a long duration, they recommend a 20% solution of Picaridin and a 20-30% solution of DEET.

There is one other alternative called IR3535. It is a synthetic substance recommended at a 20% solution.

I have since heard experts disagree with EWG and who swear that DEET is too dangerous to use. I tend to choose with caution. If you have children, do your research. Dr. Elisa Song says NO DEET, and she is a functional MD that works with children.

I will continue to use my tea tree/lavender combination essential oil, but I do intend to do more research in case I am around pets again. Please do your research and then decide what is best for you.

What else can you do to protect yourself?

- Coverup. Wear pants, long socks, long sleeves, and a hat, especially if you are out in the "wild" and even more so if you are in Lime disease, West Nile virus, or other bug-borne illness zones. Tuck the bottom of your pants into your socks. I happen to be in both of those zones, to my surprise, here in So. California.
- READ LABELS and use the lowest concentration for the length of exposure that you are expecting. Keep the bottles away from children. To put repellant on a child, put it on your hand, and then rub it on the skin of your child. Use lotion, pump, or towelette form.
- My husband suggested something he learned when he was a Marine in Vietnam. Put the repellant on the edges of your clothing. (On the bottom of your pants, the bottom of your sleeve, the collar of your shirt, the binding of your t-shirt, even on the buttons of your shirt or the zipper on your pants.) It will stop the bugs from getting between your clothing and you.

To find out if you are in these zones, check the web for:

- U.S. Map of Reported Cases of West Nile Virus
- U.S. Map of Reported Cases of Lyme Disease
- U.S. Map of Ticks Carrying Lyme Disease

When your child is at camp or when you are out camping, use mosquito nets to sleep.

Remember, the skin is the largest organ that your body has, so take good care of it. All chemicals go right through your skin and into your body.

Don't use aerosol sprays. You will breathe it in, and you can't control where it goes as easily on your body.

Test the insecticide on a small section of skin before you put it everywhere. That way, if your body reacts, you have only a small area to soothe.

Wondercide is a low toxin solution that has a spray and is recommended for both children and around pets. I found them when I was looking for a solution for fleas, which you will see further down in my chapter. I would still spray it on my hand and then rub it on my child's skin. I would apply the same way to my cat. I bought the lemongrass, but the scent was overwhelming, so you might want to try a different smell like rosemary. And yes, the brand name ends in "cide," but it uses essential oils and repels in a non-toxic way. Diatomaceous earth is effective if you rub it into your animals' fur, so I think that is a better option.

A lot of people swear by Avon Skin So Soft for a repellant. Avon says it was never intended for that purpose.

ANTS

I have a thing about ants, and they make me go a little berserk. Once they come into the house, they become pesky to eliminate. I won't buy the insect sprays; so, it has taken me a while and a bit of patience to take care of each invasion.

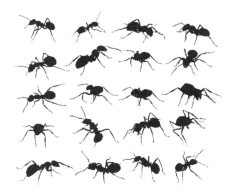

The most annoying thing is they will find one passageway into my kitchen, and if I get them to stop entering there, they immediately find another passageway. I have always had pets my entire life, so I most assuredly didn't want to do anything that would harm my pets.

I finally found diatomaceous earth. And it does a great job of stopping the ants in their tracks.

Diatomaceous earth is very effective at killing ants and other crawling insects. The Government of Canada suggests diatomaceous earth as an alternative to chemical pesticides when trying to kill ants.[121]

I buy food grade because then I know it is safe around my kitties.

The problem with using diatomaceous earth is that it is messy. I buy droppers and spray it around areas when the ants are, especially through cracks. Know that they will enter again shortly through another hole, so stay on the lookout. After a while, you will win the fight. They pick the diatomaceous earth up on their little feet and take it back to the nest.

I also make a trail around the house outside to try and keep them out. It does seem to help some as well.

I have been told that another safe ant repellant is cinnamon, sprinkled in a trail where they enter. Sprinkle the cinnamon in a wide line around your home.

One more solution. Buy organic oranges for their skin. Stuff them into a mason jar and add white vinegar. Let them soak for two weeks. Then take the vinegar and put it into a spray bottle. Viola. Spray as needed.

ROACHES

Roaches freak me out. I have only had a problem with them where I lived once in my life, and that was when I was renting a condo in, of all places, Beverly Hills.

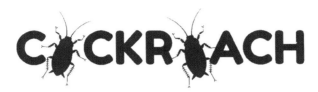

Just writing about them gives me the heebie-jeebies.

And there is a good reason for my yucky feelings about these insects. They often carry disease forming bacteria.

At the time, I was traveling quite a bit for my jewelry business. I had one roach and hadn't reacted to it before I headed out, and when I returned, there were many scampering across my kitchen floor when I turned on the light.

I did have my cats, and I had a friend living there and taking care of my kitties, but she had no idea what to do about them either.

I dreamt that I came home from a trip, opened the front door, and an entire wall of cockroaches fell out into the hallway.

I was not into spraying toxic chemicals even back then, and this was before the internet, so I went to the library and researched. I ended up buying boric acid. It worked quickly, and the roaches were gone. It's like shards of glass being digested by the cockroach, he goes back to his nest and dies. Since cockroaches are carnivorous, other roaches eat the dead roach, and then they die too.

But somewhere down the line, I discovered although boric acid is not toxic to pets, it could be. Boric acid is not as safe for animals as I originally thought.

So, if I were invaded today, I would prevent cockroaches by "putting equal amounts of baking soda and sugar out in flat containers, and they will take it.

There is a very good roach bait available commercially. It is Niban Bait, and it is made from boric acid. It would probably be easier to get this product and use it if you are in an area where roaches are very common. You can't buy Niban in stores, but it is available online. One good supplier is pestcontrolsupplies.com. When using Niban, put it under and behind appliances, around water heaters, inside lower cabinets, in the garage, and other places roaches will hide.

Keep future roaches from coming into your home by inspecting all incoming food products, all boxes, and any used furniture or appliances for the presence of cockroaches or their egg capsules. Do not store paper bags anywhere in the kitchen. Seal any holes or crevices around plumbing under sinks and behind toilets. Regularly vacuum and clean floors under the kitchen appliances. Keep all your drains closed at night to prevent them from coming up from the sewer system.

One of the best ways to control cockroaches outside is to place several pie pans filled with beer around your home. Roaches love beer, and you will find many dead roaches in the pans in the morning. And they do not check IDs. Ha! You can also put some duct tape down, sticky side up, in the house or garage where it won't get stepped on. Roaches are attracted to the glue and will get stuck on the tape."[122]

CRICKETS

Crickets are small insects that are closely related to grasshoppers. They can become a pest when they get into homes and start chirping. Controlling crickets isn't hard. Niban Bait works very well for them. It is also easy to catch a lot of them on duct tape put on the floor, sticky side up. They are attracted to the tape and will get stuck. They are important to control because they eat carpeting.

FLEAS

Non-toxic flea control can also be tricky.

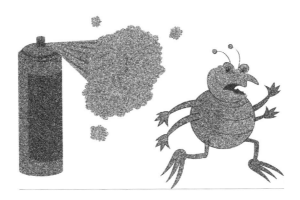

I always knew when my kitties suddenly got fleas even though they were 99.9% Indoor cats. There was always the rare episode where one of my cats made the big getaway, and then it was tricky to get them back indoors. One of my kitties escaped, and although I could hear him, I couldn't find him, and he was outdoors for several weeks. I was feeding him in the outside planter, which was high up by my front door. I could hear him at night, and the little devil would come scream under my bedroom window at night, but even with a flashlight, I could not find him. Ends up, he had dug under my backyard fence, and there was a one-foot space between my fence and my neighbors' fence, and he was hiding in there.

I finally lured him out one day with what I called "Kitty Crack," which were cat treats. I left a trail and sat down on a planter and just waited for him to come close to me, and I snatched him up. It was raining that day, so he looked like a drowned rat. (But I think he was happy to come inside again. He purred and purred like you wouldn't believe).

Well, he came home with an entire colony of fleas. I had two other cats at the time, so soon, we had a thriving colony everywhere in my home.

This was before I got an autoimmune disease, but I still did not want to use toxic chemicals if I could help it.

Use powdered Rosemary leaves as a flea and tick repellent. Dust the powder onto the pet or areas where the pet sleeps.[123]

"If you have fleas infesting your home, here is what you need to do: steam clean the carpets and all upholstered furniture. This will remove dried blood, carpet fibers, and other debris, diluted excrement, some flea larvae, eggs, pupal cocoons, adult flea feces.

Put a goose-neck lamp 8" - 10" over a pan of "fizzy" seltzer water with a few drops of dish soap at night. The fleas are attracted to the heat and carbon dioxide and drown. Sprinkle salt where animals lie; salt dehydrates the fleas, and they die.

To monitor infestations, slowly walk through suspected areas wearing white knee socks. When the fleas jump on you, you should be able to see them on the socks. Or you can put some white pieces of fabric on the floor, and the fleas will jump on them.

You can also dust the carpet with food-grade diatomaceous earth (DE). Also, dust bedding, furniture, and other areas your pets frequent. Let the DE set for five days and then vacuum it up.

Outside you can apply nematodes to your yard. You can get nematodes at garden shops where fleas are prevalent. They can reduce the flea population outside by up to 90%."[124]

SILVERFISH

Diatomaceous earth is also good to get rid of silverfish, which I occasionally see in my bathroom. You want to rid your home of silverfish because I understand that they eat your carpeting, paper, old photos, and clothing. There is no danger to humans or pets from silverfish. Just a side note, silverfish go back to the early beginnings of our earth before even the dinosaurs were here. Interesting.

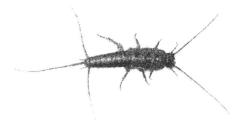

The best way to rid yourself of silverfish is to eliminate any damp areas that they might be breeding in, including under the house. Then "you can trap them by putting some flour in a small glass jar and wrapping it with duct tape so they can climb up the sides. They will get in the jar but will not be able to get out. Niban Bait is a good commercial bait for controlling silverfish. Use the fine grade Niban for silverfish."[125]

SPIDERS

Of all the insects in my area, the ones that I am most phobic about have been spiders. Until the last 20 years, I wouldn't even kill them; I would call a male friend or my husband when I had one (lucky guy) and have him get it, similar to when I was a girl, and my Dad had to get rid of the spider for me.

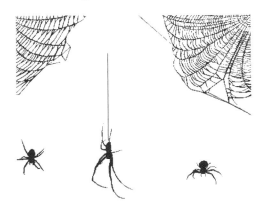

Then I moved into what I referred to as the "treehouse" up close to the Sierra Madre mountains. I rented a cute little house that was up on a second level with a storage place below it, and I was surrounded by big oak trees.

I became the queen of spiders up there. Spiders came and went on a regular basis because of the trees. And they were everywhere. I learned to live with them. And I was ok. I sprinkled diatomaceous dirt around windowsills and doorways, and cracks. I kept the areas clean so that I didn't attract bugs that the spiders would want to feed on, and I was ok. I got over my phobia about spiders.

We do have a couple of poisonous varieties here in Southern California. Sierra Madre has been known on occasion to have brown recluse. But those spiders like dark places, so I was careful before I put my hands someplace dark, or before I put on my shoes, and in the end, I never saw one.

Here in Arcadia, I have seen black widows both in my kitchen and out on my patio. They also like the dark. They freaked me out, but I dealt with them.

When I was a girl, we moved from California to Pennsylvania. It didn't help that we accidentally took a black widow with us. My Dad, a scientist, put her in a jar, and I got to watch her have her babies and then eat them. (which is why she is a black widow. Had the male traveled with us, she would have eaten him too.) Yuck. And it weirded me out.

So, being as low toxin as possible, now as an adult, what did I do? We cleaned up the area where we found them both inside and out and then sprinkled Diatomaceous earth again where they had been. Richard, the Bug Man, just told me the diatomaceous earth did nothing to keep my black widows away. If you have a stray spider, that you need to kill, use a natural product like Greenbug for Indoor.

The moral of my story is that you need to do a little research on the spiders in your area, and whether they are poisonous or not. Richard the Bugman recommends low toxin Greenbug for Indoor as the low toxin way to eliminate spiders.

PANTRY MOTHS

These insects are incredibly annoying and pesky. I think they come in flours, crackers, etc. that I bring in from the store. We had an infestation and were having a hard time killing them off. Using something toxic was out of the question around our food.

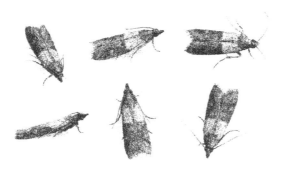

First, I bought the Pantry Moth Traps from Amazon.[126] Great reviews, but I had too many moths for them to work, and the traps caught some but not even remotely all the moths.

We planted rue and brought the flowers in and made little vases with the flowers. I can't smell them, but my hubby can. This was our first step towards success.

We threw out all the food that we thought might be contaminated with the moths. We washed down the shelves with soapy water and vinegar. Be on the lookout for larva, because those little worms are as difficult to kill as the moths are themselves. (They will crawl on the ceiling.) We put our flours and dry goods into thick plastic canisters. It was not ideal to use plastic, but better than having pantry moths all over my home. We lightly dusted the shelves with food-grade diatomaceous earth before putting the foods back.[127]

It is suggested to make sachets using mint, Bay leaves, lavender, cedar, and rue, tie the mesh bag and then place several of them around your food. It is also suggested to freeze your flours and dry goods. This cut how many moths we had, but I kept seeing new moths in my pantry, fewer but still there. What finally eliminated them was we remodeled the inside of our home. Everything was thrown away that was in the pantry, and it was refloored and repainted. The shelves were resurfaced. I haven't seen any moths since. We do keep rue in there just in case. I sure as heck don't want another invasion of the little buggers.

PAPER WASPS

Paper wasp nests are often found near doorways and other human activity areas without occupants being stung. The best way to control them is early in the Spring when they are building their nests. It is important that you knock down the nest early before the queen begins her reproduction. Knockdown the nest and then spray the area with Avon Skin so Soft. This will repel the wasps. Then get a small brown paper bag, stuff it with paper, and tie it closed. Then hang it from the area where the wasps were building a nest. They will see the paper bag and think it is another wasp nest and stay away. They are social within their colony, but they don't like their nests too close to other nests. You can hang a few paper bags all around the eaves of your home to keep the wasps away."[128]

If you don't find the nest until it is in full production, leave it alone. They don't want to interact with humans, but if threatened, they will sting. If you leave it alone, in my experience, they will leave you alone. My gardener and my assistant both ignored my advice, and at different times, they both got stung after disturbing the hive.

TICKS

You can make a good tick repellent by adding lemon eucalyptus extract to water, mix it well, and apply the mixture to clothing in unnoticeable areas, such as the inside of the pants legs and socks.

This is a great blog that I follow from a children's Functional Medicine MD about ticks and everything you need to know to keep your children safe. The Holistic Mama Doc Elisa Song, MD.

http://bit.ly/healthykidsticks

APHIDS

Make a solution of 2 cups water and three teaspoons of peppermint essential oil and spray it on the leaves of your plants.[129] Ants like the nectar from the aphids, so it's important to kill them, or they attract ants.

OTHER PLANT BUGS

Garlic Oil—Garlic is very effective in killing and repelling insects. Simmer about a dozen finely chopped cloves of garlic in cooking oil for about an hour, cool, strain it, and spray your plants. It will work on many plant pests, including whiteflies, thrips, spider mites, grasshoppers, leafhoppers, and aphids.[130]

OTHER INSECTS

There are lots of other insects that might be in your area of the country, so just note that no matter what you have, look for the non-toxic way to deal with them first. Termites, here in Southern California, react to orange oil for low toxin solution. The best method of control from a professional is with XT-2000 Orange oil. If you have a localized infestation that you can reach, then you can inject some Greenbug for Indoors into the kick-out holes in the wood. You can also do this with furniture infested by dry wood termites.

I always Google first, I talk to pest companies, I look for low toxin solutions; I ask friends and neighbors. I have always done that because I have always had pets until recently. You may have children, so you would prefer the low toxin solution. Now I look for the low toxin solution because of my autoimmune disease. My body cannot handle pesticides. And now that I know what I know about toxins, I avoid them at all costs. You should avoid them too. You can research just like I did for this chapter.

SCORPIONS

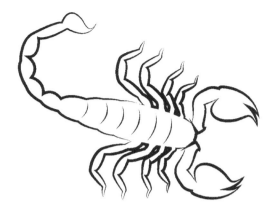

One last note. John and I bought our second home in Sedona, AZ, and yep, we have scorpions. They are in the same family as spiders, so I guess they would be considered insects. The good news is that they have a season, from March to November, so in the winter, I don't have to worry about them. There are stories in Sedona Facebook groups about encounters with scorpions inside people's homes. I have only seen one in ours, and that was when we moved in. It was in our pantry, and it was dead. They are ugly. This is the one case where we spray outside around the house. I don't know what pesticide they are spraying, but it is probably toxic. We do have ultraviolet flashlights in drawers around the inside of the house because, apparently, under that light, they glow. Since we are not in Sedona all the time, John has the pest company spray for scorpions once when the season begins. It's the best we can do. Better the toxin in this instance, outside and away from me, than the poisonous insect inside my home. It's about toxic load. Do the best that you can, and then don't get twisty.

Part VIII

Healthy Children in the 21st Century

Chapter 21

Children and Food

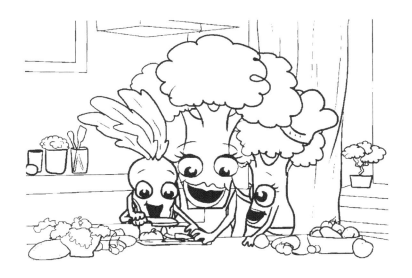

"For is there any practice less selfish, any labor less alienated, any time less wasted, than preparing something delicious and nourishing for people you love?"

MICHAEL POLLAN

THE BIG TAKEAWAYS ON CHILDREN AND FOOD:[131]

- *We, as a community, must stop feeding our children the SAD (Standard American Diet) because, for the first time, our children will NOT live as long as we will.*
- *It takes a "village" to raise a child. (An African proverb)*
- *The statistics about our children's health are appalling.*
- *Stop feeding our children processed food and fast food.*
- *"A healthy diet can have a profound effect on children's health, helping them to maintain a healthy weight, avoid certain health problems, stabilize their moods, and sharpen their minds. A healthy diet can also have a profound effect on a child's sense of mental and emotional wellbeing, helping to prevent conditions such as depression, anxiety, bipolar disorder, schizophrenia, and ADHD."*

The more I learn about toxins and our health, the more scared I have become for our children and our future generations.

I have beautiful great-nieces, and I now have beautiful grandchildren with my current husband. The statistics regarding children's health are alarming. We, as a community, must stop feeding our children the SAD (Standard American Diet) because, for the first time, our children will NOT live as long as we will, and in my opinion, this is directly related to the food they are eating. I offer, in this chapter, what I have discovered from talking to young mothers and from doing research, I intend to inspire you to clean up poor quality food, if you have children, for your children's health. This is so important, and if you are a parent and you are not aware of these statistics, I want to open your eyes.

53% of our children now have a chronic illness.

- 30% are overweight
- 16% have learning disabilities
- 11% of our children have asthma

- 10% of our children have ADHD
- 8% of our children have food allergies. There are no statistics on how many of our children have food sensitivities.
- (Although this would be important to know, conventional medicine poo-poos the concept of food sensitivities. An allergy creates an immediate reaction and can be deadly. A sensitivity starts a "slow burn" and becomes illness over a longer period. Sensitivities lead to inflammation (slow burn) Sensitivities are also known as "food intolerances," and it is estimated that 20% of our population struggles with sensitivities. My bet is, if the medical community took "food sensitivities" seriously, it would be recognized to be a much larger percentage. I have 15 food sensitivities and consider them my kryptonite. Eliminating these 15 foods from my diet gave me immediate pain relief. We need to identify them in our children so that we can also help them avoid them for their health.)
- 5% of our children have seizures
- 5% of all our children have autism
- By the time our children are 5, they can have as much as 7 pounds of chemicals in their little bodies.
- The new statistics state that millennials' health peaks at 27 and then goes downhill.
- Gen Xers make it until 37 before their health starts to decline.

  Note—The following is for everyone, but it is especially crucial for children.

GENERAL FOOD SUGGESTIONS:

1. Stop allowing your children to eat processed food and fast food.
2. You are electing to feed them for convenience and not for nutrition and their health.
3. It doesn't take that long to make meals with real live food. The benefits are enormous.
4. Cook for your children. Control what you are feeding them
5. Use quality ingredients. Eat organic. Eliminate all the toxins you can from your life and your child's life.

6. Give them real food that grew in the earth.
7. Sit around the dinner table for the years that your child is living at home. Be the example that they can follow with what you eat. Share your meals, which encourages love and community. Electronics do not belong at the dinner table.
8. Do not dictate what the child should eat or how much the child should eat. Offer choices but make them all healthy options.
9. Teach them to stop eating when they are 80% full.
10. Teach your child to be grateful for the food, for the world it grew in, for the plants and the animals that they are lucky enough to eat, and to be thankful for the people that helped get it to your table. This could be practiced in the form of "grace" or just a declaration of gratitude, but gratitude is an essential ritual for your family to practice.

"A healthy diet can have a profound effect on children's health, helping to maintain a healthy weight, avoid certain health problems, stabilize their moods, and sharpen their minds. A healthy diet can also have a profound effect on a child's sense of mental and emotional wellbeing, helping to prevent conditions such as depression, anxiety, bipolar disorder, schizophrenia, and ADHD."[132] A healthy diet will increase their ability to think and to learn. A healthy diet will help them maintain a healthy physical and mental body.

I know that a bazillion years ago when I was a child, I didn't get to choose what was served to me on my plate, and I had to eat what was on my plate before I could get up and leave the table. The concept was that children were starving in some areas of the world when my generation was little. For some, they were starving in Asia. The children that my Dad pointed out were starving in Europe. (right after World War II)

It took me years to figure out that whether I ate what was on my plate or not, the children in Europe were still starving, For years, I would move all the food around on my plate while I sat at the dinner table, and eventually I ate it, long past when I was still hungry. It's a terrible habit. My Dad was well-meaning (and a very kind man), but please don't do this to your children. He had been through the Depression when many did not have enough food, so he was going to be darned certain that I ate the food I was served.

I believe this is one of the reasons that I have had a weight issue most of my life. I didn't learn to stop eating when I was 80% full, and when I did leave the dinner table, my stomach was unhappy.

On the other hand, I was lucky. My Mom cooked and made everything we ate from scratch, so I was getting high-quality food. I encourage you to do that for your children.

Cooking is so important. As I have said in previous chapters, it's the only way you can control what ingredients you are feeding your body. It's the only way that you can ensure that your child is getting the nutrition that is important for their bodies to grow and their brains to think.

If you are feeding your children prepared foods or even worse, fast food, then you are feeding them non-food items. They are getting little or no nutrition from those foods. And you are feeding them harmful chemicals.

Cook using my "Use This, Not That" substitutions that I wrote about in Chapter 4. This list allows you to cook using high-quality ingredients. You can use any recipe using this method. When you are ready to cook, look up the recipe that you want to use on the internet, and convert it to being as healthy as possible.

When you are cooking, include veggies that would not be part of a standard recipe. Add them to everything. The more colors of the rainbow, you can feed your child, and the more vegetables you encourage them to eat is a win for your child's health.

My Mom was always adding wheat germ into everything. My brother and I hated it, and we could zoom into anything where she had added wheat germ. (We would dance a little dance "This has wheat germ; this has wheat germ. Ugh!)" She was on the right track, just with the wrong ingredient (and wheat was not drenched in Glyphosate (Roundup) in those days). Add veggies to everything you can, muffins, scrambled eggs, cakes, sandwiches, all different colors to salads, everything. Each vegetable adds nutrition and makes what you are serving healthier for your child.

All my earlier chapters on food quality matters apply when you are feeding your child. Stay away from cane sugar and fructose. Stay away from fake sugars. Stay away from low fat. Stay away from GMOs. Stay away from conventional vegetables on the Dirty Dozen list; buy those organic. More than anything, your child does not need a heavy dose of toxins with their food. Stay away from processed vegetable oils, especially if they are GMOs. Stay away from things you can't pronounce or don't know what they are. They are synthetic ingredients with no nutritional value. Stay away from factory-farmed meats and fish because they have a healthy dose of toxins, hormones, and antibiotics. All these foods are causing harm to our children.

BABIES

Let's start with the fact that our newborn infants are being born with a significant toxic load right from the umbilical cord from the mother with as many as 287 toxins right at the point of birth. Of the 287 chemicals that have been detected in umbilical cord blood, we know that 180 cause cancer in humans or animals, 217 are toxic to the brain and nervous system, and 208 cause birth defects or abnormal development in animal tests.[133] Right from the start, an infant starts with a significant toxic load directly at the point of birth. How does this impact them?

- "A developing child's chemical exposures are greater pound-for-pound than those of adults.
- "An immature, porous blood-brain barrier allows higher chemical exposures to the developing brain.
- "Children have lower levels of some chemical-binding proteins, allowing more of a chemical to reach 'target organs.'
- "A baby's organs and systems are rapidly developing, and thus are often more vulnerable to damage from chemical exposure.
- "Systems that detoxify and excrete industrial chemicals are not fully developed.

- "The longer future life span of a child compared to an adult allows more time for adverse effects to arise."[134]

I have been listening to a symposium on the liver, which is our detox organ. If the body cannot detox all the chemicals out of the body because of overload, it "protects" the body by tucking the chemicals and poisons away in the body's fat and bones. The chemicals hide there until they begin to leak out, making the body's organs increasingly unhealthy later. It's so crucial that you eliminate the toxins before you feed them to your child, at any age.

If you are planning to have a family, clean up your toxic load first. You should be eating organic, avoiding GMOs, and using low toxin products for some time before the point of conception.

This approach is important for the father as well as for the mother. You should be eating real live food and eliminate anything from your diet that you cannot pronounce or do not know what it is. (like natural flavors) You are what YOU eat, and unfortunately, your newborn also inherits what YOU eat.

The comment about a father's diet is from a new study, which even surprised the researchers. "Folate-deficient diets in the male rats in the study made their children more likely to have birth defects and altered genes associated with chronic diseases like diabetes, obesity, and cancer."1[35] How can this be? The father's diet had an impact on how his genes expressed in his sperm.

We are learning all of this through the study of Epigenetics, which is still in itself, in its infancy. But it is known that diet and lifestyle do impact how the tendencies we inherit in our genes are expressed, so it makes sense that this is essential information for both the soon-to-be mother and the soon-to-be father before conception.

Give your child a clean slate at birth and give it an optimal chance for good health and to develop its body, mind, and natural intelligence by living and eating low toxin.

I just listened to Michael Skinner, MD, and Jeffery Smith of the Institute for Responsible Technology. They were on a podcast. And it was rather surprising.

No one has ever studied the multi-generational impact of Glyphosate. Dr. Skinner is part of a group from Berkeley that just finished a multi-year study into this. What they have found so far is worth noting. There is no impact of Roundup on the first generation and little on the second generation, but the impact on the third generation is horrific. This means that what you eat before you conceive that child impacts your great-grandchildren even more than your children. Many of the Moms died in childbirth in the third generation, and the impact on the sexual organs and the kidneys of third-generation children was huge amounts of disease and infertility.[136] 90% of the third generation had disease issues.

We don't even begin to understand the damage that eating all this Glyphosate is having on the human race.

I also learned today that there are 40,000 lawsuits against Monsanto now for creating cancer in people who have been exposed. And yet, it is still being sprayed on our crops.

As a responsible parent, it is increasingly clear that becoming low toxin long before conception is important for the long-term health of your child.

BABY FLORA

There is a difference in baby flora depending upon whether the child is born vaginally or from C-Section. If the baby is born vaginally, they get all the healthy probiotics of the mother. If they are born C-Section, they do not. A child that is vaginally born receives a boost to their immune systems, and it protects their intestinal tracts.[137]

Babies born via cesarean section (C-section) don't have that same advantage.

"Now, a new procedure that levels the playing field is starting to get some attention in the medical profession.

"It's called vaginal seeding.[138]

"The process involves wiping down a baby—who is born via C-section—with gauze that has bacteria from the mother's birthing canal. The hope is that it will expose the baby to the same bacteria as if they were born vaginally," according to Mary Lou Kopas, chief of midwifery at the University of Washington's Medicine Northwest Hospital Midwives Clinic.

"The point of vaginal seeding is to give the benefits of normal bacteria and flora," from the mother like vaginal birth, she explained to Healthline.[139]

There are some risks involved with vaginal seeding, so if you choose to do this, have a robust conversation with your doctor. A fair number of mothers have a staph infection that could be transmitted to the child.

Babies born via C-Section tend to have more problems breathing and tend to suffer from asthma more often that children vaginally born. Being birthed through the vaginal canal squeezes all the liquid out of the baby's lungs.

Children that are vaginally born get breastfed more quickly than C-Section infants. The mother has less recovery time from vaginal birth.

You probably know that if possible, you should breastfeed your baby. Again, this only makes sense if you have significantly lowered your toxic load. There are many advantages for the baby and you. Mother's milk builds the child's natural immune system and contains antibodies that help your baby fight off viruses and bacteria.[140] A mother's breast milk has all the vitamins, nutrients, calories, and fluids that the infant needs to be healthy.[141] There are also health benefits for the mother to breastfeed.

The advantages of breastfeeding your newborn are numerous for you and your baby:

- New findings have concluded that upwards of 30% of beneficial bacteria found in a baby's gut comes directly from a mother's milk. What's more, an additional 10% comes from the skin on the mother's breast.[142]
- Mothers breast milk is nature's perfect infant food.
- For your newborn infant, the milk gives them immune-boosting antibodies.
- It passes healthy enzymes to the child that scientists have not been able to replicate

- Its easily digested by the child
- It is easier for your infant to utilize the breast milk causing less stomach upset, diarrhea, and constipation for the child since it is custom designed by nature for the child.
- It reduces the risk of viruses, including ear infections in the child, and lowers respiratory infections.[143]
- There are fewer cases of SIDS in breastfed infants.[144]
- It protects the child from getting some diseases in later life.
- The fatty acids in breast milk are thought to be the brain boosters. So, although it is currently being studied, feeding the child breast milk may give the child a higher IQ.[145]
- Breastfeeding shares love and bonding with your child.
- Breast milk helps your infant sleep better and encourages healthy circadian rhythms in the child.[146]

However, if you cannot breastfeed[147] (or if you choose not to) feeding the child an "off the shelf" formula is probably not a wise option. "Most commercial formula options, even organic ones, contain ingredients, additives, and preservatives that aren't good for the baby."[148] Formulas are loaded with chemicals and are often also soy-based, and 95% of soy is GMO.[149]

If this is the case, there are some other options. You can make a homemade option that is nutritionally healthier for the baby than any manufactured formula. One possibility noted here is from Weston A. Price, and the other is from Wellness Mama.

> https://www.westonaprice.org/health-topics/childrens-health/nourishing-a-growing-baby/
> https://wellnessmama.com/53999/baby-formula-options/

If you aren't breastfeeding, you won't get the good bacteria transfer from the mother, or the incredible bonding between mother and child that the child would receive from breastfeeding, but at least you are not feeding your baby an inferior formula that will increase their toxic load and even possibly leave the child nutritionally deficient. Some of the bonding can be overcome by bottle-feeding the baby and maintaining the skin to skin contact.

Some Mom's cannot breastfeed, and that isn't something to get twisty about. Your baby will feel that, and their tummy will respond to those emotions. Hold the baby close with skin contact and love and choose one of the healthy options above for feeding.

Moms try to make the best choices they can for their children. Do your research, make informed decisions, and don't stress over decisions you made in the past. John's mother (my husband) worried for years because of a physical condition that prevented her from breastfeeding her children. The additional stress impacted his mother and his siblings.

The next step, of course, is what do you do once you wean your child off breast milk or your homemade formula. Again, baby foods are loaded with synthetic ingredients and chemicals, and foods that are not optimally healthy for your child. This starts somewhere around 7-8 months, and again food should be home prepared.

The best blog that I found on how to feed a small child is *Nourishing the Next Generation* by Beetroot.[150] She gives a step by step guideline as to how she started feeding her baby new foods and how to get her child to eat real food as the food her baby could eat progressed. I strongly recommend that you look up her blog and read it. Other Moms that I have talked to have introduced foods a similar progression.

In the beginning, you pulverize the food so that it is the consistency of jarred baby food. All the mothers have emphasized that you should offer new foods in small quantities along with foods that you know that your child likes and will eat. You just put it on their plate. You do NOT insist that the child eats it. Each day, you continue to offer the food until one day it does get eaten, and then you start by introducing another new food.

Beetroot Brooke offers multiple selections in small quantities on her child's plate and then lets the child choose what they want to eat. All options are nutritious.

I have also learned that children respond positively to food if you make it fun. Bright colors, fun patterns made with nutritious food all promote healthy eating.

I have found fun bowl mats with the bowl in the shape of a frog or an animal, and different compartments made from silicone that encourage happy eating.[151] There are duckies and bears and elephants made from silicone. Do NOT use plastic as it is toxic, but silicone is safe.

You will also want to be creative with how you lay the food out on the dish. Google fun food for children on Pinterest, and lots of boards come up with great ideas to make food fun.

I have also found superfood powders in intense colors that I use to make inventive recipes. I believe in eating all the colors of the rainbow. The company is Unicorn Superfoods out of Australia. http://bit.ly/unicornsuperfds, they have a cookbook with ideas and a fantastic Instagram page loaded with great ideas.[152] Shipping is included in their price, and it comes quickly. It's a win, win, win. These are bright colors that add nutrition and additional flavor, and that your child will want to eat.

Since I am always talking about eating the rainbow, I have fallen in love with these superfoods. I am planning a cookbook with a focus on eating the rainbow recipes since each color has unique gifts for the body. Cooking with color feeds your child what they need to grow up strong, and color improves their brainpower; it also makes the child WANT to eat the food because it is more fun (and tastes yummy).

You want to raise your child with the ability to make choices; you want to control that the choices are all good for them. Only keep healthy options in your home.

This does not change as the child progresses through different food cycles and eats more real food. Feed the child what you, the adult, is eating. Vary variety and color, shape, and texture on the child's plate. Your child will mimic you.

Multiple Moms that I have talked with have suggested teaching the child to read labels as early as possible. My husband says that children are little pitchers, what you pour in and what the child observes from you, becomes a lifelong habit for them.

More than one Mom has expressed that as she is in the store reading labels, her child is mimicking reading labels even before they can read. They will pick up the can or the box and let their little finger slide across the ingredients on the package. Once they do learn to read, they will learn what good ingredients are and what harmful ingredients are. These children are instilled with good eating habits right from the beginning, and these children are more difficult to sway once the child is finally on his own and off to school.

One Mom shared with me that when her child was offered an unknown food, the child brought it home to discuss with her as to whether or not they should eat it. The child is not perfect, they did eat pop rocks at a birthday party, but in general, they are proud of making great choices when they are away from their home.

If the child eats something that is off your program, don't get twisty. Remember that it is all about "toxic load." Just have a conversation with the child as to what healthier options might have been.

This mother also shared that a year ago, her mother was not as concerned with healthy food choices when her children stayed with them. The 3-year-old told her mother, "Grandma, we don't eat that." Wow. Now a year later, they have influenced Grandma so much that only healthy choices are offered. It can be done. And it doesn't mean that the food is not delicious while it is also nutritious.

This is what Beetroot Brooke writes in her blog: "I think some people believe August (her son) and kids like him are missing out on a piece of childhood, but that's because, as a society, we've come to prize sweets and treats and the pleasure food brings, over robust health and vitality. We need to redefine what makes a great childhood. It's no longer about having a coke bottle with a straw, cotton candy at the baseball game, or Gatorade at the basketball game. It's about experiences: unforgettable family trips, getting outdoors to get hands dirty in the garden, and quality time reading books at bedtime. People are strapped for time, so slowing down to do meaningful things, like prepare real food and have undivided attention for our children, have gone to the wayside, which is why they are like *gold* now."[153]

People ask me all the time if John and I are deprived since we don't eat the SAD (Standard American Diet). We were deprived BEFORE we started feeding our bodies what we needed to return to health.

Limit sugar and refined carbohydrates in your child's diet. Sugar is addictive, so limit what they get to eat. Sugar impacts every organ in the body negatively, so stay away as much as possible. Refined carbohydrates turn to sugar, and therefore are not healthy.

Children are eating *34 teaspoons of sugar a day as kids.*[154] Our body wasn't meant to handle more than two teaspoons of sugar a day, so you can imagine how harmful this is, all by itself, to a child's body.

Teach your children why you are feeding them the food they are eating. Encourage them to ask questions about their food. Teach them where food comes from and then how it gets on the table for them to eat. Encourage them to ask questions. Don't dictate as they get out into the world, teach them the advantages of eating real food, and allow them to follow the example of how you eat and teach them the why. As your child grows older, you want them to be able to make their own decisions, and you do not want them to feel deprived. The more they understand how you are feeding them, the more likely they will choose to eat that way. Bring up your child to be the leader of the pack that eats healthy food. Bring them up to be a superhero.

Encourage your child to cook with you. Partner with them to make their lunch plans and have them make up their lunch box with you. I have a chapter coming up for your child to garden with you. Make them a part of the process of eating healthy food. And always make it fun. Set a joyful expectation of eating real food.

BREAKFAST

Breakfast does not need to be complicated. You could boil some eggs on the weekend and grab them for a quick breakfast during the week. Make overnight oats in the fridge and have it in small, easy to grab jars. Add different fruits and nuts to their porridge in the morning. Have your child help you as much as possible. Enroll them in making and serving their food.

It's not hard to make homemade granola. The advantage is that you control that you use organic oatmeal, and you can cut the sweet way down. I use organic nuts and ghee and then sweeten with a touch of maple syrup. I use Ugly dried fruits, which encourages recovering food waste. (I don't use their dried peaches since peaches are on the Dirty Dozen list, but I do use their dried apricots and dried kiwi). And I use Enjoy Life chocolate chips, which are 69% chocolate and soy-free.

I recommend Vital Farms eggs. Their chickens are out foraging for their nutritious food, which then passes to their eggs. They get to eat grass and berries, and they get a change of scenery regularly. This makes for happy chickens and healthy eggs. And yes, they are a few cents more per egg, but they are worth it. (We also think they taste better.) Why is it important to eat eggs from humanely treated chickens (other than the obvious, that it's better for the bird?) Its essential for you and your children's bodies as well. They aren't passing their stress hormones on to you through their meat and their eggs.

If you are using dairy milk, make it full fat. Remember, your child doesn't have to have dairy for their health, so this is if you choose to serve it to your child. Same with dairy yogurt. Full fat is much healthier for them. For a full explanation, see my chapter on dairy in my first book, **It Feels Good to Feel Good, Learn to Eliminate Toxins, Reduce Inflammation, and Feel Great Again**.

If you are serving almond milk, make it organic. There is a law that almonds get "pasteurized" to kill viruses, and usually, the manufacturing method is to do the process with a chemical related to formaldehyde. You don't want that in your body or your child's body. Organic is steamed at high temperatures to meet the law requirements.

SNACKING

Make sure that the options that they get to eat at home are nutritious, wholesome, and easy to grab. Keep veggies cut up in the refrigerator for snacking. Keep a variety of fun dips available for the child to dip the veggies into.

I just found Kite Hill Almond Sour Cream. Yummy with Simply Organic onion soup mix. (Primal Palate also makes great spice mixes for dips.) John and I were like two little kids eating this. Fantastic and it tasted like the old chemical onion soup and sour cream dips but is way healthier.

 (I have been told dips are big with kids.) Keep a variety of different hummuses, nut butters, dips, etc., that are wholesome and healthy available. Make your own; it's not difficult and so much healthier. Look for Paleo or vegan recipes. Variety is important. Make homemade vegetable chips from a variety of different vegetables. Slice them thin and then crisp them on low in the oven. I stir melted ghee onto them in a bowl and then add our favorite seasonings. You are going to want a couple of great slicers to get veggies thin for chips or dips. http://bit.ly/diffslicers You can also buy shapes, like stars and hearts, to cut up your veggies for serving. (Again, make it fun.) If you own a dehydrator, then use it to make crispy real veggie snacks.

Aim for good protein and fats in the snacks you keep on hand. Save fruit for dessert for dinner.

Other healthy snack ideas:

More Snack Ideas for Children (and Adults)

- Plantain or sweet potato chips with guacamole—Make your chips. It's easy if you have the right mandolin (slicer). (see above) If you do buy store-bought, make sure they use a healthy oil and that they are organic. Make your guacamole; it's easy. I make mine the fast way, avocado smashed, with fresh tomato salsa (mild) from Whole Foods and lemon juice. I add organic powdered garlic and onion and viola. All good. All healthy.

- Trail mix—I save jars. Since we use ghee instead of butter, I use the ghee jars for a variety of purposes. Trail mix is easy to make up and keep on hand to grab & go—almonds, pecans, cashews, large coconut flakes, organic raisins, dried cherries, pumpkin seeds are some of the items I add to the mix. (I soak my nuts before dehydrating them)/ or I purchase already sprouted organic nuts. I also use Enjoy Life chocolate chips to add variety to my mixes. I have recently found soy-free white chocolate morsels from Pascha with rice milk. Yum.
- Homemade crackers—I have a blog with recipes on my website at https://cherylmhealthmuse.com. There are also some great new organic and healthy crackers available on the market.
- Pitted olives—are an excellent choice for snacking.
- Hard-boiled eggs—Vital Farms sells them in packs, and their eggs are pastured and organic. Portable. Filling. Versatile. Need I say more? Worth the money. See above.
- Cucumbers, snap peas, or carrot sticks, celery with homemade ranch dressing—I use Danielle Walker's recipe. http://bit.ly/dwalkerranchdressing, It is nondairy and healthy, and as close to buttermilk ranch that I can mimic without the chemicals or the dairy.
- Lately we are also using Primal Kitchen salad dressings, all healthy ingredients, all tasty. Primal Kitchen has many salad dressings now that are yummy and clean—Perfect for dipping and all real food ingredients.
- Tortilla chips w/ guac or salsa—I prefer Honest Jackson's organic Tortilla chips when I can get them since they are soaked in lime juice and makes the grain easier to digest. But if I can't get that, I get an organic brand. I also love Siete[155] brand.
- Popcorn—Buy organic and pop your own. There are also many store-bought popcorns available that are organic and good. We enjoy Quinn popcorn. We also like Lesser Evil and Buddha Bowl popcorns with sea salt. We buy this kind of snack from Thrive Market to save money. There is a membership fee that I immediately make up with the savings from buying my hard goods from them. (And they deliver. What's not to love?)
- Pretzels—We enjoy Quinn, and we also like Newman's organic pretzel sticks.

- Larabars—For an occasional on the go treat. Watch sugar amounts on the label as they vary.
- Enjoy life—has protein chocolate balls, and rice milk crunchy chocolate bars, which are a great occasional treat. They also make yummy seed and nut bars.

Ok now, what do you do for lunch? For the first years of the child's life, you are controlling his options. As he is old enough to leave the house, it gets a little more complicated. I know some Moms are concerned that their child will be eating unhealthy snacks and foods that other children have with them.

I follow a mom on Facebook who is doing an outstanding job at communicating what ingredients are healthy and what ingredients should be avoided. She is gotten very famous going after Big Food for toxic ingredients in their processed foods, and she has gone after fast-food companies for the same reason. She is having an impact.

I wrote on my Facebook page one day that I would prefer that you stay away from anything you can't pronounce or don't know what it is, like natural flavor, than to go after the fast-food companies. She responded that she is concerned that when her child goes off to school, she won't be able to control what her child is eating. Her approach is to change food to be healthier as it is made. She is taking on Big Food. A valid concern and a worthy approach, but it is dealing with the big picture and not specifically what her child will confront and then choose.

I have discovered from the moms I have discussed this with, fingers crossed, the child can be prepared to deal with this and make healthy choices. Not being a mother, maybe I am naïve?

"It's not what you do for your children, but what you have taught them to do for themselves that will make them successful human beings."

ANN LANDERS

I suggest you knight your child as a Jr. Veggie Ranger™, as you send them off to school to be an emissary for healthy eating. Instill in them the pride of eating delicious, healthy food. There is a company that has a slogan "I eat delicious, nutritious and never suspicious."[156] Make your child proud that they eat this way.

More thoughts:

1   No plastic. Not their plate, not their juice or water bottle, not their sandwich bag. Use bamboo utensils. Plastic leaches poisons into their food, and it's simply not worth it. Plastic is loaded with poison.
2   Buy them a stainless-steel water bottle to carry to school.
3   What do you put their food into then? A stainless-steel lunch box.

Recommendations:

https://www.planetbox.com/collections/spare-parts

http://bit.ly/lunchboxsiliconestainless (they are promoting recipes with peanuts and peanut butter which you should not pack for your child who could be around other children that have severe allergies.) They also have silicone separators and cups if you go to their website.

http://bit.ly/allstainlesslunch for an all stainless set of 3 lunch containers.

You can buy stainless steel containers for hot chocolate and hot soup. (Make your own hot chocolate with alternative milk and real cocoa. Sweeten with a touch of maple syrup, coconut sugar or honey).

The key is that you don't want plastic touching the food. Silicone lids are great. Stainless steel boxes are great. I would be careful of the collapsible silicone boxes (I had a couple of accidents with mine when they collapsed suddenly with food in them), and I think it would be impossible for a child.

4   Concentrate on high-quality protein and good fat. If you need a refresher on this, check my first book, It Feels Good to Feel Good, Learn to Eliminate Toxins, Reduce Inflammation, and Feel Great Again.
5   A good healthy lunch should be balanced. Include:

- A protein: Applegate lunch meats, pastured chicken, leftover grass-fed beef from the night before, pastured turkey.
- Veggies: organic, in all colors, in small pieces. Easy to pick up and eat. Include at least three colors in the assortment.
- A healthy dip for the veggies
- Fruit: cut into small pieces
- Make protein or fruit kabobs. Consider wooden skewers (break off the sharp points) with the colored veggies and the fruit. It makes them more fun.
- A Carb: organic: popcorn, potato chips, Pretzels
- Mix up shapes and colors. I own small cookie cutters in heart shapes, star shapes, butterflies, and flowers. I use them to cut veggies into fun shapes.
- Use all the rainbow colors

Benefit:

Control your child's nutrients. Avoid processed foods.

Eating high nutrient food improves learning.

Sweets should not be everyday treats, but that does not mean that you should eliminate them completely. When I bake, I often will choose items to bake from Danielle Walker's cookbooks. She uses clean ingredients, and the items that I bake from her recipes are amazing. Her "Real Deal" chocolate chip cookies would rival my Mother's Toll House cookies of the past. I use Enjoy Life chocolate chips because they are soy-free and 69% chocolate. I also love her Walker Shortbread cookies, and when I bake a pie using one of her recipes, they are out of this world. The crust is from cassava flour. There is no need to buy processed treats that are loaded with GMOs, chemicals, and obnoxious ingredients. Even better, teach your child to cook with you. Build memories that will fondly carry with them into their adulthood.

The important thing is to feed your child for nutrition. The body wants to be healthy; you need to give it the right building blocks. This is even more important for a child. Choose foods for their nutritional value and teach your child to love them.

Make bone broth regularly and keep it on hand. Make sure you are using pastured animal bones. If the animal has eaten a lot of chemicals, the chemicals lodge into their bones. Bone broth is healthy for you and your family. It's not hard to make. Chicken and turkey are the easiest. You can then make bone broth into a variety of soups loaded with veggies either as veggie soup or pureed as whatever the veggie is that you added to the broth. I love to make cauliflower soup. I steam it, throw it into my Vitamix, add my bone broth, ghee, seasonings, and I have a nutritious, fast, delicious lunch or first course. There are many fine bone broths now available for purchase. Careful of the ingredients in them. Avoid caramel coloring.

https://healthykidshappykids.com/2016/11/27/nourish-family-bone-broth/

Dinner should be together around the dinner table, whenever possible, as a family. Not only is this a great time to be an example of good eating habits, but it's also a wonderful time to bond and find out about each other's day. I have great memories of sitting around the dinner table with my folks. They both had a great sense of humor, and family stories were often told repeatedly to great delight. We shared our wins and our defeats and got advice about how to regroup when necessary. I have very loving memories of my childhood as a result of our dinner meals. Just writing this now makes me smile. We always ate at 6 pm, but whether it's 7:00 or 7:30, it should be a time when the entire family is home to share the meal. We were not allowed to watch tv during the family meal. You should not allow electronics at the table.

Buy clean meats, which means the animal should be pastured and that he has eaten his natural diet. We eat grass-fed grass-finished beef. Pastured chicken. Heirloom pastured pork. Bison and lamb both graze on grass. Yes, these meats are more expensive, but you don't need large quantities of these meats. For an adult, the portion size should be the size of the palm of your hand. These animals have not been given hormones to make them grow faster, and they have not been given tons of antibiotics to keep them alive until they can be butchered and then land on your plate. They have been humanely treated, so they are not loaded with their stress hormones. Trust me; you have plenty of stress hormones of your own. These meats provide small amounts of goodness to you and your child's body. Dr. Mark Hyman, a functional MD that I follow, suggests that meat should be a condiment to accompany the veggies that you are serving on your plate.

Three-quarters of your plate should be vegetables. Try for at least three different color groups. Each color has a gift, and together synergistically, the colors provide health. Buy organic, especially if the fruit and veggie are on the dirty dozen list.

Remember that food quality matters. Staying aware of what you are feeding your child will help you raise disease-free children who are productive and healthy.

Keep in mind that even depression starts in the gut. A happy gut is a happy mindset for your child.

Last comments—there are so many allergies and sensitivities now, that as a parent, you need to observe what happens to a child's body as you introduce new things into their environment. This includes foods, fabrics, medicines, pets, etc.

For an explanation of the differences between sensitivities and allergies, please check out that chapter in my first book **It Feels Good to Feel Good, Learn to Eliminate Toxins, Reduce Inflammation, and Feel Great Again**.

It's also important to remember that at an early age, when given healthy foods, children tend to gravitate to what they need at the time. Let them make their own choice; I want to reinforce that all the choices should be healthy.

Chapter 22

Children and the Outdoors

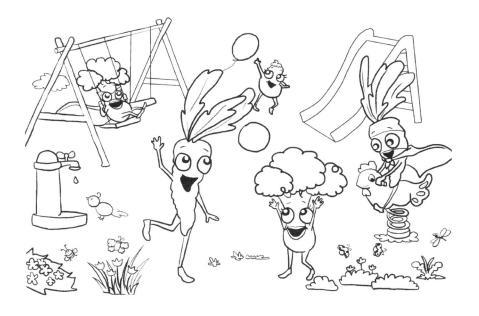

THE BIG TAKEAWAYS ON CHILDREN AND THE OUTDOORS:[157]

- *Our children have been coined "The Indoor Generation" since 90% of their time is spent indoors.*

- *We need to allow our children just to be, and to enjoy exploring the great outdoors, which could happen in a city or country living.*

- *A lack of daylight is impacting our children's ability to learn, increasing their blood pressure, and causing depression in 15% of our kids.*

- *Air is most polluted in children's rooms and is five times more polluted than the outdoor air.*

- *Let children play in the dirt. Let them get dirty. Let them play in the mud. The microbes that they get from dirt are good for children.*

- *Plan fun activities to get your child outdoors and then afford them the freedom they need to enjoy it.*

Our children are not getting exposed enough to the joys of being outdoors and the health benefits that come with being in nature. They have been coined "The Indoor Generation" since 90% of their time is spent indoors. A lack of daylight is impacting our children's ability to learn, increasing their blood pressure, and causing depression in 15% of our kids. To make it worse, the air in our homes is poor quality, and it is most polluted in children's rooms and five times more polluted than the outdoor air.[158]

This has become so serious, that outdoor words from years past are being eliminated from dictionaries to make room for new digital words. "In 2007, Oxford's 'Junior' dictionary, for children age seven and above, tossed out several words from the natural world. Words like 'moss,' 'blackberry,' and 'bluebell' were erased from Oxford's dictionary for children in order to make room for technological terms like 'blog,' 'chatroom,' and 'database.'"[159]

I just bought a magical book for our grandchildren on Amazon called "The Lost Words"[160] Anansi International; First Edition (October 2, 2018.) It has become an international phenom to bring enchantment back to lost words for children.

But beyond words, I don't want children to lose the outdoors in any way, most of all in reality.

When our children do get outside, everything is scheduled. They seem to go from activity to activity, whether it's soccer, baseball, ballet dancing lessons, art, or some other activity. We are keeping them very busy in their off-hours and not allowing them to just be and to enjoy exploring the great outdoors, which could happen in city or country living.

"Blame it on our smartphones and increasingly tight schedules, but in the United States, we're spending less time outside than ever before. Nature deficit disorder has become a legitimate diagnosis, as the average American spends 93% of their lives indoors. According to one poll, 70% of moms in the United States remember playing outside every day as a child, but only 26% of them can say the same of their kids."[161] Other countries are placing a greater priority on encouraging their children to spend time outdoors, and are seeing the benefits of that policy.

Nature has many gifts for our children. We need to be encouraging our kids to explore these gifts. It could be as simple as letting our young children play on equipment in a local park. Let children play in the dirt. Let them get dirty. Let them play in the mud. The microbes in the dirt are good for them.

Since I already wrote in chapters (19 and 20) about why returning to nature and why forest bathing is so important to the health of adults, I wanted to emphasize that the outdoors and nature are just as important for our children to experience, if not more so. Let's explore what the benefits are for children to be outside.

In one article I read, the subject of raising a "wild child" was being encouraged. (Within reason, of course.)[162] Our children, today, lead very supervised lives.

"Kids need nature; they need unstructured time, and they need play. It may seem like this is just 'fun,' but we know from research that this is how they grow and properly develop."

Nature has benefits for us all. We slowdown in nature; we live in the present moment when we are outdoors; the outdoors takes us back to our roots, and it helps all of us understand more about the world around us. Being in nature impacts our mood, lowers depression, soothes and reverses stress, and improves self-esteem. These are all things that should be learned early in life.

There are real physiological and psychological benefits of being out in nature. Furthermore, movement increases brain power, so getting children out into nature improves their learning. Being out in nature, being able to go out and climb trees, swing, and hang upside down are all things that improve motor growth development, and they also improve learning when the child enters school.

As adults, we often do not prioritize downtime, and in the long run, that is not healthy for us. We all need downtime, and our children need it too. We need to encourage unstructured downtime for children, which is time for them to rejuvenate and relax, and nature provides this kind of opportunity. Encouraging your child to get into nature and have unstructured time teaches him that this should be a priority throughout his life.

Another advantage of a child getting out into nature with other children is that they get to figure out things for themselves. It encourages them to become problem solvers. They may not do it right, but that's even more important when they are young when the risks are low. As we know, as adults, making mistakes is part of the process for finding success. Learning tenacity for problem-solving is an especially valuable skill to learn. Kids learn to adjust and approach the problem from different points of view until they finally get over the hurdle. Invaluable.

Kids learn limits when they are out in nature. They are supposed to jump on and off things. They pick up branches and whack things. This is all normal behavior. But there are limits that they learn as well. They should not hurt themselves or others while they are whacking things with that branch, and they pick up what is and isn't acceptable quickly. If kids are continuously supervised, they never get to learn these boundaries on their own. Kids need to learn self-regulation. Through trial and error, kids learn self-confidence that they can handle themselves. "You cannot promote confidence without letting kids take risks," says Aliza Pressman, Ph.D. "They can learn so much more about being a competent adult by going through the obstacle course of being outdoors and wild play."[163]

Small children adapt easily to nature and outdoor settings. Being outdoors fosters creativity. They are naturally curious about their world, and there are many wonders for them to explore outdoors. It doesn't need to be complicated, just sitting and playing in the dirt can bring moments of complete pleasure. Gathering leaves can bring a small child joy.

Children who play outdoors have stronger bones because their bodies naturally produce Vitamin D. They sleep better because of playing outside. They become physically stronger because of movement. This sends blood to their brains and helps them to learn faster.

A child that plays outside has their senses awakened "to the sight of birds and butterflies, the smell of flowers and trees, and the sounds of water rushing or leaves rustling. Importantly, they get a vital break from their intense indoor, too often digitized, and highly regimented lifestyle."[164]

Being in nature activates more senses. Your child can see, hear, smell, and touch outdoor environments. This increases their entire human experience.

Encouraging an older child to leave his electronic screen, computers, games, phones, etc. and go into the great outdoors will take a more creative approach. Screen time is an easier choice, but the child will have a wider perspective and grow more if he can step outside.

Let's explore ways to get your children into the great outdoors.

There is a website called Ranger Rick, run by the National Foundation of Wildlife. They have articles, magazines, and games all to promote a better understanding of nature for your child. They have a magazine and a book club all geared to your child's enjoyment of nature.

Ranger Rick has many suggestions for the outdoors so that you get out into nature with your child. The natural world is fascinating to you child. So, don't miss this opportunity for spending loving time exploring with your child. The times you spend with your child outdoors will be loving memories when your child is grown.

One of the things the Ranger Rick people encourage is gardening for wildlife. I am going to discuss gardening for the child's food in another chapter, but here let's explore how wonderful it is to grow plants that attract butterflies and bees that the child can see out his window and out in the garden. My husband's first wife gardened for butterflies, and it was charming to be out in the flowers that the butterflies loved the most. Her garden got certified as an official wildlife habitat for butterflies.

Start having a daily "green hour" with your child. "The idea of a 'green' hour comes from research on creative play and health by the Centers for Disease Control and the Academy of America Pediatrics. Research shows the best way to connect young people to a lifelong concern for nature, wildlife, and the outdoors is through regular positive experiences."[165]

"The American Academy of Pediatrics and the Centers for Disease Control agree an hour of free play and moderate activity daily is a prescription for lasting health. Increasing a child's time in nature and the outdoors does not have to be a heavy burden for parents and caregivers; a quick stop at a local park on the way home from school, fishing in a local stream, or an impromptu picnic outside all count."[166]

Other things you can do to get your children outdoors.[167]

- Join with other parents in the neighborhood and set up treasure hunts. Make a list of things that your child can "hunt" for. Make a short, simple list of things for your kids to look for outside—such as "a shiny object" or "something you can hold a liquid in." The satisfaction of finding the objects turns it into a reinforcing activity, and it will keep them outside in search of the next list item.
- Buy your children's books with pictures and send them outdoors to identify things. I had a tree finder book that I dearly loved when I was a child. I could sort a series of clues until I had identified the tree. You could do something similar with birds, bugs, leaves, trees, or flowers from your local area. Buy audible tapes of bird calls and let them identify what bird is making the song. These adventures are like treasure hunts. I know I was thrilled as a child when I was able to identify something.

- Buy them (or even better help them make) a special box to keep their outdoor "treasures" in.
- Buy them a magnifying glass.
- Get them a microscope so that they can see things up close that they collected outdoors.
- Encourage the child to look up at the stars. My father had a rudimentary telescope, certainly not as high quality as are available today, but I loved going outdoors and finding Jupiter or Saturn or the Pleiades (seven sisters). Just looking at the craters on the moon was a thrill. And the joy of doing this was something that I shared with my Dad.
- Buy them a small shovel to dig in the dirt. Buy them gloves and a garden trowel. Let them play in the dirt and even better, let them play in the mud. This is all pure delight for a child.
- Take your child to your local parks, especially if they have outdoor performances. Plays, music, puppet shows are all magical for a child.
- Start a collection with your child. It could be fall leaves, or rocks, or shells from the beach. Make sure if you are in a public park that you are allowed to take whatever you are gathering. These things would be great to keep in their "treasure box," and then they can add to their collection.
- If your child is "hooked" on electronics and reluctant to get outdoors, buy them an inexpensive camera and teach them to take photographs or let them record videos on your phone. This way, your child creates a photo/video log of all the adventures the two of you go on together.
- Take them on a hike somewhere in your local area. It could be in the woods or along a riverbank or on a trail that leads to a waterfall. You could take them to a lake and let them fish. Check out my emergency pack of food that I keep with me and carry your healthy snacks. Make sure that you take breaks, and if possible, carry a fun book to read to your child when you slow down and sit.
- Go on an adventure to pick flowers and leaves and then teach your child to press them when you both return home. Collect rocks to paint. Encourage them to find natural objects in nature that they can use creatively.

- Build something with them. It could be a hummingbird feeder or a bird feeder, or boxes to grow plants in. Encourage them to build with you. They will have such pride in the projects that they do with you.
- Create a fire, in a fire pit, and cook your food on it and then have a picnic.

It would be great to walk every day in the woods, but if this is not possible, take a break in a local park. Walk the dog together. The important thing is to get outside and enjoy it together, or to send them off with their friends to enjoy the outdoors.

Form an outdoor club with your friends, neighbors, and family and plan an outdoor activity once a month. Put it on your calendar. Depending upon where you are going and what you are doing, buy books to explore what kinds of activities will be available and what kinds of animals might be seen. Do this together in preparation for your outing. Make it a fun excursion long before you go on this adventure together.

Getting teens outdoors with you is likely going to be more of a challenge. Parents need to limit the amount of time that their teenagers are in front of a screen, be it a tv screen or a computer screen. Outdoor activity is very healthy for children.

No doubt, spending more time reading and doing homework increases achievement in school. However, time spent outdoors increases social conditioning, which is also important for the child.

Suggested activities to get your older child outdoors:

1. Kite flying

   It develops the mind as well as the physical body. Kite flying is challenging and very rewarding. If you did organize a neighborhood community for outdoor activities when the child was younger, now that they are teens, you can run friendly kite flying activities with your neighborhood group.

2. Biking

   Take your child on a cycling excursion. Include his buddies. The exercise would be good for all of you. Teach your children the rules of the road and bicycle safety. Make sure that all of you wear helmets.

3. Hiking

   Invite your child and his buddies to go hiking. It could be a daytime excursion or overnight, depending upon where you live. Hiking into a "wilderness" area and enjoying all it has to offer is important to get your child excited about living an outdoor life. Choose your area and read up on what it has to offer. You could hike in and then fish or learn all about the ecological things in the area. The more you know, the more you could make it very interesting for your child and his friends. Make sure that you follow the local rules and customs. Teach good stewardship by policing your trash.

4. Stargazing

   Buy a telescope and invite your child's friends over for an evening of stargazing. Equipment is much more advanced than when I was a child. You will probably want to get maps as to where the constellations are now in the sky, but new telescopes also have functions that tell you all that right from the telescope. Read up on the stars that you are going to be viewing with your children and their friends and talk knowledgeably with them on the subject.

   Some of my best memories are stargazing with my Dad. He had a rather basic telescope, but he would always focus on the Pleiades, which are, to this day, my favorite stars. I rarely go out a night that I don't look up, and if it is clear enough, I find the Pleiades and count them. I can't always see all 7 of them (it is now understood that there are more than 7 in the cluster, but seven are most readily seen), but I have very warm feelings towards them and count, however many of them I can see. It makes me smile and brings back fond loving memories of my Dad.

5. Take a river trip

   Be the "cool" parent and take the children on a river trip. It could be on a raft, or in a canoe. Check out the areas where this might be available. Most teenagers would be enthralled to go on a river trip with their buddies.

6. Dodge Ball

   I recall watching a hilarious movie about Dodge Ball years ago. Rent the movie and then find a court where you can supervise a game of dodge ball for your children and their friends. You will all have a "ball" (a wonderful time), and it will be an unforgettable experience. Don't forget; you will need the appropriate equipment and the right type of ball.

7. Buy a frisbee

   Once you have the frisbee head for the park with your child. This is fun to do just with your child or with a group of your child's friends. If you have a dog, they will enjoy the outing as well.

8. Buy a Hula Hoop

   Its incredible exercise, if you have 2, your kids can have contests of who can go the longest. It's a hoot and another experience that they will remember.

9. Get outside and walk.

   You could get outside and walk the pet, or you could hoof it with your child and walk to the store, but whatever the motive is, walking outside will do your teenager a ton of good.

10. Find the right outdoor activity for each child

    If you have more than one child, don't hesitate to schedule an activity with each of them so that you have alone time with your child outdoors. Talk to your child about where their interests are and pick the activity that you do with each child based upon that conversation. As your children grow older, they will develop different interests. It's wonderful to enjoy one on one time with each of them anyway, and all of you will enjoy your activities more if they are tailor-made.

Final thoughts. It's always good to explain to your child WHY it's so good for them to spend time outdoors, whether it is in the back yard, or on a more extended trip. I know I always enjoy things more when I understand the "why," and children do as well.

Chapter 23

Teach your Children Where Food Comes From - Garden with your Child

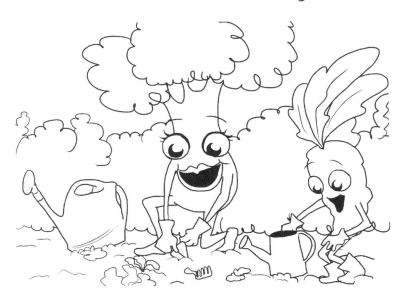

THE BIG TAKEAWAYS ON TEACHING YOUR CHILDREN WHERE FOOD COMES FROM:[168]

- *Our children are confused as to where the food they are eating is grown.*

- *We have lost contact with the origin of our food.*

- *Our children do not understand what meat comes from which animal.*

- *30% of our children don't know that most cheese comes from cow's milk.*

- *Food quality matters. We are what we eat, but the basic problem is that we have no idea what we are eating.*

- *Big agriculture is not concerned about our health. Big Agriculture is concerned about their profits.*

- *We are not eating "food." We are often eating "food-like substances."*

- *Our government is not subsidizing "healthy food." Frankly, they are subsidizing "unhealthy food."*

- *YOU are responsible for understanding where your food is coming from and what you are putting into your body and your children's bodies.*

- *You have a much better chance to raise children to eat clean, healthy food if they understand what it is, where it came from, and how it is grown.*

About two years ago, I came across an article in the Washington Post that stated that 7% of our population believed that chocolate milk came from brown cows. It made me stop and think. At first, I thought it was ridiculous, especially when I realized that that was 16.4 million adults, slightly more than the Pennsylvania state population. I realized that we have a problem. The Innovation Center for U.S. Dairy released the results of this online survey, and they felt it showed that Americans don't have any idea where their food is grown and raised.

The most attention-getting stat was that 48% of people surveyed didn't know how chocolate milk was made.[169]

A portion of the American public is not educated about the origin of our food. "The Washington Post writer Caitlin Dewey pointed to a USDA study that showed that nearly one in five adults were unaware that hamburgers are made from beef. Even more, people were unaware of the standard size of U.S. farms and what farm animals eat. The study noted there seems to be no difference in agricultural education among economic class and race."[170]

Other astonishing statistics—"U.S. Department of Agriculture found that 12.3% of people surveyed in Missouri and Indiana thought that hamburger was made from the meat of pigs, and 5.9% didn't know what it was made of."[171] (Kansas, next door to Missouri, is the third-largest producer of cattle/beef.)

In 2011 a group of elementary children in California had no clue that pickles came from cucumbers.[172] Mind you, California is my home state, and we grow more food for the U.S. than any other state. 30% of these same children had no idea that most cheeses were made from cow's milk (remember California is the state with "happy cows.") And these children had no idea that much of the food they were eating was processed.[173] They also did not know that onions and lettuce were plants. Four in 10 didn't know that hamburgers came from cows.

"Another study, published in the Journal of Agricultural Education, showed that 72% of children living in urban California don't know that cheese is made from cow's milk. Further, a 2017 study published by Michigan State University showed that 48% of Americans rarely or never seek out information regarding the origin of their food. In other words, it's not just chocolate milk that Americans are confused about."[174]

In yet another study, "15% of children believed chocolate and cucumbers are grown on trees.

"One in 20 even falsely believed that avocados are laid by animals.

"Proving that society is failing to lay down the foundations for basic food knowledge, almost a quarter also thought turkey, chicken wings, and sirloin steak come from a pig."[175]

John and I drove out to see our rancher in Sedona last Christmas to buy our pastured organic beef, and in our conversation with our rancher, he commented that when his wife went to nursing school, someone asked her what she did for a living before she decided to become a nurse. She commented that she and her husband were ranchers. One of the young nursing candidates commented that she would only purchase her meat from a grocery store because then no harm was done to the animal. What? Yikes. Where did she think that packaged beef came from?

There appears to be a great deal of confusion about basic food facts. When I was young, I learned this in elementary school. But even though we lived in a populous area of Pennsylvania, Bucks County, I still was not very far away from farms, and we would visit them. We would go to an Amish farm to buy meat. We would go to strawberry farms in New Jersey to pick strawberries. I would then help my mom wash and stem them and get them ready to be frozen so that we would have berries all winter. My Dad was an engineer, so I certainly wasn't working on a farm, but I was aware of where my food came from, how it was grown, where animals were raised, and I was a lucky girl because my Mom cooked.

We, as a population, have moved further away from the farm, and more of us are living in cities. We have disconnected from our real food. We are choosing convenience over real live vegetables and fruit, and we are eating processed and fast food. (And as a result, we are choosing convenience over health as well.)

We are not cooking, so we are not controlling what we are feeding our bodies and feeding our children. This is becoming a huge issue. I have stated earlier in this book that 53% of our children have a chronic illness. I just read that 60% of Americans have chronic illnesses. It's all connected. We need to start to show and teach our children where their food comes from, and we need to make what we feed them a greater priority. Food quality matters. We are what we eat, but the basic problem is that we have no idea what we are eating.

"How did we become so disconnected from the sources of our bread, beef, cheeses, cereal, apples, and countless other foods that nourish us every day?[176] Two hundred years ago, Americans knew where their food came from, largely because they were growing it themselves. We evolved, over several generations, to a place where eating food and producing food were different and segregated experiences."[177] We need to bring food back to where it belongs—at the center of our families and communities.

"So much of the food entering the marketplace is being modified, over-processed, and lowered in quality, and it's happening faster than you can bring a fork to your mouth."[178] Unfortunately, none of this is making our food more nutritious. In most cases, it is creating food with little or no food value at all.

Let's think about what big agriculture means to our food.[179]

1. Big agriculture is not concerned about our health. They are in the business of making large profits no matter what the cost is to our health.
2. Knowing what the animals you eat are eating is important. What they eat is what you eat, and if they are fed low-quality food and GMOs, you are eating the same. Also, you are eating the added antibiotics and the added hormones that the animals are eating to mask that they are unhealthy.
3. There is a correlation between what we spend on food, and how much it costs, and it is related to how much more we are now spending on health care. No wonder more than half our children have a chronic disease, and as adults, we are in the same position.
4. In many cases, we are not eating "food." We are eating "food-like substances." We are eating manufactured synthetic ingredients that have little, if any, nutritional value. Your body wants to be healthy, but you must feed it ingredients that allow it to do its job. You have read what I have written earlier. Garbage in, garbage out. If you don't eat quality ingredients, your body cannot rebuild its cells, as explained in my "Food Quality Matters" chapter.
5. Our government is not subsidizing "healthy food." Frankly, they are subsidizing "unhealthy food." YOU are responsible for understanding where your food is coming from and what you are putting into your bodies and your children's bodies. Start with a campaign to educate your children where food comes from and encourage healthy food eating habits.

So how do we teach children where their food comes from? You have a much better chance to raise children to eat clean, healthy food if they understand what it is, where it came from, and how it is grown. There are several ways of going about this:

1   Take your children with you when you shop for real food. Take them to the grocery store and the farmer's market.
2   Make friends with your farmer and visit his farm. Take your children.
3   Go to the ranch and purchase your meat. Talk to the rancher and understand his commitment to health.
4   Take your children to pick fruit in season. In Southern California, you can take them apple picking, pear picking, and cherry-picking. Let your kids get their hands into the dirt. You probably have some local fruit growing in your area. Research and take advantage of what is available in your area.
5   Google UPick Farms. I see several states that have them. Look for Birthday Parties at the Farm, Pick-Your-Own Produce, Educational School Tours, not to mention special harvest festivals, and many have farm-to-table dinners at the farm.
6   Look for places where you can watch cheese get made. The first time I saw cheese being made was in Tillamook, Oregon. There is also a place in the Seattle Pike Street Market where you can watch cheese being made.
7   Explore Public Markets like the Seattle Pike Street market because they may have other foods you and your children are not familiar with. I used to love to see the Geoduck clams that were in the open market there. They are fascinating and quite delicious and create quite a bit of humor, just seeing them. (Look them up. *smile*)
8   When I lived in the Seattle area, we used to go clamming. What a fun excursion that was. We would look for little holes in the sand and then dig like crazy. When we got the clams home, we would soak them overnight so that they would spit out their sand, and then steam them for dinner the next night.
9   Take your children fishing. If there are trout in your streams and rivers, take them trout fishing. If you live close to an ocean, take them saltwater fishing.

10 If you live in New England, you can take a licensed boat and help catch your lobster.

11 In Louisiana, you can help catch your crawdads.

12 There are also catch and cook programs around the United States. In Louisiana, you can catch and cook game fish. In Seattle, you can catch and cook salmon. In British Columbia, Canada, you can catch and cook Sturgeon, and wow, are they big.

13 Take your child to a county or state fair and visit the farming exhibits.

Explore what is available in your area.

Teach your children to garden. You have several options here. You can till and plant a small plot in your back yard. You can buy a tower and garden on your patio. You can grow herbs in your windowsill. Let your children have the joy of planting seeds and then watching the fruits of their labor. They will be thrilled to eat food that they have had a part in growing.

It's hard to imagine where food comes from unless you've been in the trenches digging holes; planting seeds, bulbs, sprouts, or seedlings; then, watching these living things grow into full-fledged plants that kids can pick and eat.

These are some fun and easy projects to get you started:[180]

1. Buy organic celery. Cut off the stem. (Eat the stalks. They are great for dips or nut butter as an after-school snack.) Place the celery bottom in water. It only takes a couple of days to start to grow roots. You can then take it outdoors and plant it in the dirt. You could also plant it in a container on your patio.

2. Plant your garlic cloves in a little dirt. You need more patience for this one, but they will eventually start to grow. You will get long spears like chives to grow, which you can clip off and use on meats and salads for flavor.

3. Make a terrarium in a canning mason jar. Take a little plant in its little pot, put it into the lid of the mason jar, and then screw the jar onto it. Viola!

4. Grow herbs in the window of your kitchen. Have your children make herb vinaigrette and herb butter with the new growth.

5. Buy different soils, and have your little ones, ages 3-8, make mud pies. They will love getting their hands muddy, and it's good for them. Teach them to observe whether the mixture stays together (clay) and can be formed into shapes, or whether it becomes all crumbly. (sand based) For instructions go here: http://bit.ly/makeamudpie

6. Throw a gardening birthday party. Ages 2-10.[181]
   a Start with making homemade invitations. Cut out pictures of plants, flowers, garden tools, seed packets, and give your child a glue stick and paper to make the invitations.
   b The decorations for the party should be fresh flowers and vegetables. Munch food should be easy to hold. Serve pieces of veggies and fruits of all the colors of the rainbow with different kinds of dips.
   c Activities would include painting a pot and planting it with some small plants.
   d They could also plant some large seeds like pumpkin seeds to take home, and you would explain the excitement of waiting for the seed to sprout.
   e For games and other possible activities, go here: http://bit.ly/gardenpartygames
   f Instead of cake, make cupcakes using almond flour and coconut sugar, and make the tops look like flowers. You could even use edible flowers on top.
   g "Read a Garden Story: If things get too wild, settle things down by reading aloud the inspiring and wonderfully illustrated children's book, Miss Rumphius, by Barbara Cooney. It tells the story of a woman who, to fulfill her grandfather's directive to make the world a more beautiful place, decides to do so by planting lupine seeds wherever she goes so that all can enjoy these beautiful flowers."[182]
   h Get little clay pots, put bathroom paper cups inside and fill them with dairy-free chocolate pudding or chia pudding. Let them "eat dirt." Make almond flour chocolate cookies to crumble on top (low sugar) and have an organic gummy worm on top.
   i For party favors, start with Oriental Trading and see what's currently available. Right now, they have some garden party boxes that are

very cute. http://bit.ly/orientaltradinggardenparty They currently also have some very cute flower stickers. Then make up little bags with seed packets, little gardening gloves[183], little wheelbarrows[184], little red wagons[185], little watering cans[186,187], And since it is a party, include organic worms. http://bit.ly/organicworms. Let your child know that these are not everyday treats. (sugar)

7. Kitchen scrap gardening. I am sure that you know that you can put toothpicks into an avocado seed, put it over a glass with the bottom touching water, and it will start to grow a mini avocado plant. But did you know that you could do scrap gardening with lots of other scraps? You can take the seeds of citrus and plant them (and yep, they will grow). You can take cut a 1-inch piece of carrot, and its top will grow. Put it onto pebbles. You can also do this with a scooped-out top of pineapple again on pebbles until it starts to root. You can do this with lettuce, basil, fennel, cilantro, onions, and more. Make this a fun project to do with your child.[188]

8. Finally, you could try tower gardening. I know Juice Plus sells a tower that you can plant and have fixings for your salads at any time of the year. I just read some people have them in their living room. Although I don't recommend Juice Plus itself, because I want you to eat the whole real organic plant, I love the concept of their tower, and it would be a great way to grow veggies with your children.[189] There are also inexpensive greenhouses available that might work. During warmer times of the year, depending upon where you live, you could do real backyard gardening with your children or join a community garden.

My suggested rules to teach children to eat are simple. So, let's figure out how to educate our children about food and help them discover the importance of the quality of their food and reading labels.

- If you read the label and you don't know what an ingredient is, don't eat it.
- If you can't pronounce an ingredient, put it back on the shelf.
- Eat only foods that will eventually rot. You can keep a McDonald's hamburger for years on your counter, and it's in the same shape as when you purchased it. Yuk.

- Processed foods have preservatives, dangerous trans fats, loads of sodium, and sugars. Teach your children to avoid those ingredients.
- Only eat meat that has eaten well, and that has eaten his natural species-specific diet. You are what it eats. Eat pastured organic meat. If the animal you eat has only eaten genetically modified and heavily sprayed grains with herbicides and pesticides, then the ingredients you are eating are the same and laced with poison.
- Eat organic. You do not need a heavy dose of poison with your food.
- Eat all the colors of the rainbow, from a farm as close to you as possible. Buy produce that is in-season when the nutrients are prime, and the food is in abundance so that it is more affordable.
- You must cook. If you don't know how to cook, take a cooking class. Go with your child and go with a girlfriend. Make it fun. Cooking is one of the nicest, healthiest things you can do for your body and your family. I have sweet memories of cooking with my mother. Leave your children a legacy of cooking too.

These are fun things to do with your children that will have long term health effects. Teaching them where food comes from is important. Having them participate in growing their food and then eating it, builds an appreciation. Teaching them to cook and having them enjoy the joy of eating home-cooked items is priceless. And trust me, they will remember it for the rest of their lives, and it will serve them well.

Chapter 24

Read to Your Child

"Children are made readers on the laps of their parents."

EMILIE BUCHWALD

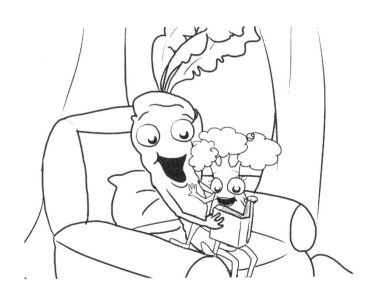

THE BIG TAKEAWAYS ON READ TO YOUR CHILD:[190]

- *If you can encourage your child to be a reader, they will have a greater understanding of the world around them; they will have a larger vocabulary; they will perform better in school; and they will be able to entertain themselves where ever they are, in any part of the world, because they have a book or a Kindle.*

I decided that this was an important chapter to include in my book because it is about the brain health of our children. It is also commonly agreed that readers become more successful in life.

If you can encourage your child to be a reader, they will have a greater understanding of the world around them; they will have a larger vocabulary; they will perform better in school; and they will be able to entertain themselves where ever they are, in any part of the world, because they have a book or a Kindle. They will have better alone skills. They will be better intuitive thinkers. It helps them develop better "concrete (The Doer), analytical or abstract thinking (The Analyst), logical thinking (The Orator), imaginative (The Inventor), and creative (The Original Thinker)"[191] thinking.

I was an avid reader from the time I was 7. (It all began with Nancy Drew books.) Even then, they were dated, but that amused me. To this day, I use slang from those books that I love, like "swell."

I believe that I have learned more about the world because I have been an ardent reader, and reading has significantly increased my enjoyment of life. It has taken me to places in the world I would not have otherwise visited. "It has allowed me to see the world through a character's eyes. Watching a character interact with the world around them is powerful."[192] It has taken me to times in the past so that I could understand them, and the experience of people living in these times became more intimate. Reading about a character "in history" is completely different from reading a series of dry historical facts in school, and it was so much more enjoyable and memorable. You understand the time that you have stepped into completely differently, and you can taste, touch, and feel that historical time in a much more intimate fashion. You are, in your mind's eye, standing next to that character in that timeframe, and you are experiencing what they are experiencing with them. It's magical.

"When you read fiction, you can be someone you'd never otherwise have the chance to become—another gender, another age, someone of another nationality or another circumstance. You can be an explorer, a scientist, an artist, a young and single mother or an orphaned cabin boy or a soldier, or a detective like Nancy Drew."[193] Fiction allows you to explore a different time, a different culture, a different technology, a different place, a different personality, a different relationship to others and gives you a fresh perspective. It develops empathy with the characters we are experiencing. And when you put the book down, you are changed from having had that experience. You understand the world differently, and it has enhanced your life.

Reading has also soared my imagination into the future and allowed me to explore possibilities.

"Reading fiction not only develops our imagination and creativity, but it also gives us skills to be alone."[194]

Reading is physically good for us. It reduces stress, improves sleep, increases self-care, it's good for our minds and our hearts. It gives us a break from whatever is happening in our own lives and takes us to another place. Readers tend to have a less cognitive decline in later years. Readers tend to be more inclusive of people different than themselves. And it gives us a greater understanding of animals and the need for their well-being.

Reading gives us crucial skills for interpersonal relationships. And reading gives us different skills for handling different people and different situations.

Both fiction and non-fiction add value to life and learning that helps develop who we are and who we will become.

Non-fiction books help us discover things we do not know. They offer us real-world solutions to the problems we are facing. Learning to read with factual books as well as storybooks is a way of preparing children for life. Children are naturally curious, and they love to discover new facts about their world.

"Everyone can agree that reading is an important component in developing a successful life. Consuming content sharpens your intellect and builds your knowledge set. It seems almost universal that the more successful you are, the more you read."[195]

I was one of those kids that was at the library every week, checking out the maximum number of books allowed and reading them under the covers with a flashlight at night. I loved reading so much; I was an English Lit major at UC Berkeley. Although I will admit, I read so many novels in a condensed period in college that for a while, it almost killed my joy of reading. But I was reading novels like **War and Peace**, in addition to multiple other great works, all at the same time, and I was never without a book. I read on the bus on my way to school; I read between classes; I read on my breaks during the job that I did during college, I read over breakfast, lunch, and dinner. I read continually to keep up.

My husband shares my joy of reading, and it is something that connects our souls. Even though he is a mathematician and a statistician, his minor in college was literature, and he reads more than I do. We don't share a love for the same genre of books, but we do both have a passion for reading. (John is wild about fantasy and science fiction. I am wild about historical novels, and espionage, or detective stories.) We both have curious minds and read nonfiction.

One of our guilty pleasures is to listen to books on tape as we drive between LA and Sedona, where we own homes. The eight-hour drive becomes completely enjoyable because we listen to audible books. It not only makes the drive palatable, but also is something we look forward to, and if we haven't finished the current book we are listening to, it's the pleasure of seeing the old serials at the movies back in the '30s, and the 40's when we continue with the book. We get another installment in the story. (I belonged to a youth group that played those serials during the summer, and I fell in love with watching them too.)

So, this chapter is about how do you foster a love for reading in your child? You need to be reading to your child from the point of conception into their teenage years.

READ ALOUD TO CHILDREN

Repeat after me; reading should be all about pleasure. If you teach your child to enjoy the experience, then you have won more than half the battle for them to be lifelong readers.

During the time that you are expecting, it is important to sing, play music, and talk to your unborn child. "Talking, reading, and playing a variety of music can help stimulate baby's senses and improve her brain development."[196]

The best time to start to read to your child is in the third trimester before birth. Experiments, where the mothers read the same passages over and over again to their unborn child, got immediate reaction from their infant once it was born, and they read the same passage. They can hear and take comfort from their mother's voice, and they look forward to bonding with their mother and hearing her read the moment they are born. Some great books to read to your unborn child can be found here. https://www.greenchildmagazine.com/reading-to-unborn-baby/ and here https://preemiemomtips.com/books-to-read-to-your-unborn-baby/

"Then, continue reading to infants as soon as they are born! Use rhyming books, such as Mother Goose rhymes, and songs to help with language development. 'Rhymers will be readers.' (*Reading Magic*, pg. 85.) There are many more do's about reading to children than don'ts, as it's simply most important just to read!"[197]

If a parent reads aloud to their child early and often, then the letters and words will naturally come into the child's world.

The parent must make the words they are reading mean something to the child. Make the reading enjoyable and fun for your child. "According to Mem Fox,[198] there are three secrets of reading: being able to make the print mean something, understanding the language, and our knowledge."[199] These are great books to read to infants to toddlers and beyond. https://preemiemomtips.com/top-10-baby-book-ideas/

Reading builds a connection with your child, especially at the end of the day. Reading to them is a very bonding experience. It allows them to share emotions with you that might otherwise be left unsaid. When they are old enough, let them pick the book, read it to them and then ask them questions about why they choose that book. Let it be the gateway to understanding what your child is feeling and thinking at that point in time. Let the book be a gateway to the pleasure of a good story and a greater understanding of your child for you.

And I found this interesting. If that child cannot pronounce a word, don't make them struggle with it. Say it to the child clearly, and then move on. You might want to return to the word and say it clearly again, but don't allow the child to struggle with the word. That will lower their enjoyment of the reading experience.

There are two types of reading. The first is auditory; the child hears the story as it is read to them. Auditory includes looking at the pictures and discussing what they show. As your child grows older, reading becomes visual, they "read" the story. But auditory continues to be important at any child's age, from pre-birth to teenager and should be continued in the home.

I remember when my brother and his wife read **The Chronicles of Narnia** out loud to my niece, Amy. She was enthralled with the story and fully engaged. The beauty of CS Lewis's book series is that it works on a variety of levels. It was a wonderful fantasy world for children; it was an allegory for adults, and it dealt with religious philosophy for those who could catch it. This makes it a fully satisfying book for all. I know that they read it again when they had a second child, Rachel, some years later, and they all enjoyed the book series one more time.

Reading aloud to kids has clear cognitive benefits. For example, brain scans show that hearing stories strengthens the part of the brain associated with visual imagery, story comprehension, and word meaning. One study found that kindergarten children who were read to at least three times a week had a "significantly greater phonemic awareness than did children who were read to less often." And the landmark *Becoming a Nation of Readers* report from 1985 concluded that "the single most important activity for building knowledge for their eventual success in reading is reading aloud to children."[200]

Reading aloud may support students to develop sustained attention, strong listening skills, and enhanced cognitive development.[201] Reading aloud makes a huge difference by the time a child is in kindergarten with an improved ability to listen.

Reading to very young children is linked to decreased levels of aggression, hyperactivity, and attention difficulties.[202]

- Start early
- Read often
- Sometimes read the pictures first with your child before you read the story[203]

Once you are reading the story, make correlations to the child's life and get them to talk about it. Whether the character is someone like someone else in the child's life, whether the character in the book likes something that the child likes, whether the character in the book is going on an adventure that the child has experienced, or wants to experience, use the story as a way to get your child to talk about himself, his own experiences, his loves, the people in his life and his emotions.

Children will also benefit from hearing the same story numerous times. I am not a parent, but my friends and relatives who have children all had a book that was their child's favorite, and that story was read over and over and over again. It ends up that this is a beneficial behavior. And remember, reading should be all about pleasure. This is a list of books for your infant to toddler and early years that make kids laugh. Kids like to read funny books! A whopping 70% of kids say they want books that make them laugh, according to Scholastic's Kids and Family Reading Report. https://www.pbs.org/parents/thrive/fifteen-books-to-get-the-whole-family-giggling.

This concept does not change as the child grows older. Children who were 17 still looked forward to books that made them laugh.

I have collections of **The Far Side** and of **Calvin and Hobbes** because I still love to laugh from books.

The consensus seems to be that when the child begins to read more on his or her own, parents should continue to read out loud with them and to have the child read out loud to the parents. Their vocabularies continue to grow, and their reading out loud skills, like pronunciation, continue to grow as does their confidence in reading out loud.[204]

Suggestions for being successful at reading out loud to your child.[205]

1. Let your child pick their book as soon as they are old enough to do so. Find a way that the books are stored with their cover side out. Build low shelves that the books can stand up on or screw rain gutters onto the wall that can hold the book cover side out. Children respond to fun, bright covers, and it makes it easier for them to identify their favorites.

2. Leave books in every room in your house. (See my note about cover side out above). Take books everywhere you and your child go—to the park, to the dentist, to the doctors, to a friend's home. I am never without a book at my ripe old age, and you don't want your child to be either. It allows a child to entertain him/herself everywhere.

3. Read the child wordless photo books when they are young. This is a way for both you and your child's imagination to come alive. As you turn each page, ask questions.
   - What do you think is happening here? (comprehension)
   - What makes you think that? (inferring)
   - What do you think will happen next? (predicting)

4. Why? (vocabulary and oral language)"[206]

5. In the beginning, start with small books. This makes it easier for your child to concentrate on the subject in the book. You can always choose another small book to read with your child if they are asking for more.

6. Use your voice to make the story interesting and to be creative. This makes it interesting for you and fun for your child. Make sound effects, change voices for different characters. Make appropriate noises to sound

like animals. Lower your tone if the subject is sad or scary, speed up your cadence if the subject is happy or gay.

7. Continue to read aloud to the child as they grow older. The more pleasure you and your child can get from reading loved books together, the better your child comprehends reading and will thrive in a classroom environment. You should be reading to or with your child well into their teens.

8. Don't stop every 2 seconds to explain a new word. Explain a word and then move on. The next time you read this book with your child, you can explain a different word. What is important is to maintain the pleasure of the story with your child. The more they find pleasure in reading, the more likely they will enjoy reading later on their own.

9. Make a literary meal with your older child. Many books have food as the storyline, like Split pea soup from **George and Martha** or spaghetti and meatballs from **Cloudy with a Chance of Meatballs**.[207] Anything that you can do to make books come alive for your child will serve them well.

10. Make reading and books a part of dinner conversations. Ask about what the child's favorite book is. Encourage the child to be inventive and tell a story to the family. (If you look back at my chapter about children and food, and the importance of eating dinner as a family, this is part of the ritual that will be remembered for life and reinforce good habits and attitudes in your child.

11. Encourage storytelling time after dinner. This is a great list of ideas to get your children telling stories and enjoying the process. This would not replace reading to your child, but it is a marvelous new activity to encourage creativity and language skills in your child. https://www.thebookchook.com/2011/06/sixteen-sensational-storytelling-ideas.html

12. A PBS suggestion is to create a reading tent in the living room. Only allow your child into the tent when they want to have a book read to them. It doesn't have to be fancy, but it does need to be playful and comfortable.[208]

13. By the time the child is 7, they will have developed some reading skills of their own. Take turns reading but keep the ritual alive of reading out loud. You can take turns paragraph by paragraph or chapter by chapter but continue to do reading aloud as a special time with your child.

14. Connect books to real life. If your child loves dinosaurs, take them to a Natural History Museum. In LA, we have a great display of dinosaurs, and we also have La Brea Tar Pits. If your child loves trains, take them on a train ride. In LA, you can take a little train at Griffith Park, and you can take a longer train ride there. You can visit Thomas at a train museum in Orange County. My point is, your area will have something different, but take your child to whatever that is and make the book come alive. If you have a little girl that is enamored with dancing, take your child to the Music Center or a local dance studio. Or take her to one of the American Doll stores around the country. A little girl's pure delight.

15. Get your child a library card. I was a permanent fixture at our library, starting at about 8. I would wander around and read book flaps and then decide what I wanted to check out. I understand children still prefer physical books, or they can put themselves on the list for kindle books when they come available.

16. Libraries also have wonderful events. Authors come to libraries to read their books to children, and there are groups that children can join to discover new books and new genres.

17. Take your child around the library and read the signs for the different sections and explain what they mean to your child. This will encourage your child to explore when they are older and on an adventure at the library alone.

18. Don't forget graphic novels where the child learns to read the pictures to know the story. There are appropriate graphic novels for children to enjoy. Check out this list—https://www.readingrockets.org/booklists/graphic-novels-read-pictures

When searching for new books to read to your child, look for funny books, and look for books that show diversity. Both are so important for health and empathy.

"89% of kids ages 6 to 17 agree that the favorite books 'are the ones that they have picked out for themselves.' And book choice starts early, as 67% of parents with kids up to age 5 reported that their kids choose the books for read-aloud time. This goes up to 81% of parents with kids ages 3 to 5."[209]

Great site with book suggestions for all ages. https://www.readbrightly.com/

Reading with your child will bring you and your child beautiful memories and what better gift can you give your child than the joy of words and books.

Chapter 25

Water Safety for Children

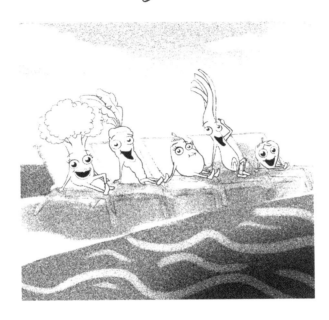

Swimming Safety—Important Facts to Be Aware Of:[210]

Drowning is the leading cause of accidental death among children one to four-years old.

Never leave your child unsupervised in or around a pool or any container of water. When you and your children are around water, never let your child out of your sight for more than a few seconds at the most. Tips to protect your child:

- Always make use of children's floatation devices. Be aware your child could still drown even using these devices if left unsupervised.
- Learn CPR. Make sure your class included child CPR. Check with the American Red Cross for classes in your area.
- If you have a pool, have a well-rehearsed plan to deal with a drowning emergency.
- American Cross also often offers swim classes for the entire family. They start at six months. Taking a class with your children reduces the risk of drowning by 88%.
- For children under the age of 4, keep children in water that is shallow enough for them to stand.
- Make sure you have a fence around the pool on all sides that is at least 5 feet tall.
- The gates should have locks that self-close. The latch should be at a height that children cannot reach.
- Running in a pool area should be forbidden.
- An adult should always be in arm's length away from any young child.
- One adult should always be present that can perform CPR.
- An approved life vest is far more secure than inflatable swimming floats. The float seems secure but does not protect your child.
- Be prepared, Keep a shepherd's hook, a life preserver, and other rescue equipment near the pool with easy access.
- Keep a telephone close, but not near the water. It is electrical. Keep the phone where you have access to it, but where it is safe to be stored.
- Forbid young children to jump or dive into the pool.
- Never let children swim alone.

- Make sure that children wear proper apparel.
- Impress upon children the seriousness of the pool. No games, consideration always, No pushing others into the pool.
- When swim time is over, remove all toys from the pool. This way a child won't be tempted to go into the pool alone to play.
- When pool time Is over, secure the pool so that children cannot get back into it.
- For every child that drowns, there are five children that are treated in an emergency for near drowning.
- 75% of the children that drown are boys.
- After use, empty blow-up pools.
- No tricycles in the pool area.
- No electrical appliances near the pool.
- No running should ever be allowed in the pool area.
- It is the law to have a fence that completely surrounds the pool. This will protect your child and neighboring children from entering the pool area.
- Fences should be too high to climb. No objects should be close to the fence that could help a child climb over the fence. It should be 4 ft high at a minimum. The fence should have no footholds or handholds to help a child climb over it. Chain link fences are a bad choice because of the ease of climbing.
- The gate must have a working self-closing and self-latching closure. It must open away from the pool. Latches should be 54" or higher.
- The door to the pool area should have a loud alarm.
- There is also an alarm that you should install that is on the sides of the pool under the water. This alarm detects movement.
- If the pool is above ground, avoid steps and ladders. Remove these when the pool is not in use.

At a party, designate an adult to be the "watcher." Make them a bright badge so that they are easy to spot.[211]

Part IX

Our Beloved Pets and their Health

Chapter 26

Introduction to Pets - Pets and Toxins

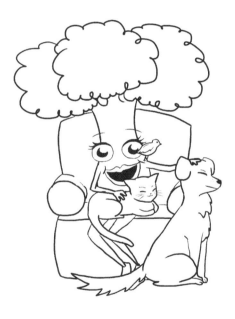

THE BIG TAKEAWAYS ON PETS AND TOXINS:[212]

- *The FDA has, for decades, allowed the pet food manufacturers to violate Federal law.*

- *An estimated six million dogs and nearly six million cats will be diagnosed with cancer this year. The experts that I have been listening to and reading believe that 90% is due to environment and lifestyle, and only 10% is genetic.*

- *1 in 1.65 dogs will succumb to cancer. And 1 in 3 cats. Your dog is four times more likely to get breast cancer than you are, eight times more likely to get bone cancer than you are, and up to 35 times more likely to get skin cancer than you are." However, over-vaccination remains rampant, lawn chemicals are frequently used, and our food is sprayed with even more chemicals as it is being grown. The chemicals that we have around our pets are over-the-top toxic.*

- *We have a reactive health care system for humans and our animals. We need to change to a proactive system.*

INTRODUCTION

This subject is very personal to me.

While I was researching for my health after I got sick, it didn't occur to me that the toxins in my life were also the toxins in my pet's lives. As a result, I lost all 3 of my cats to cancer, one at 12 and one at 14, and then one year later, my red-haired boy, Beeper, who would have attached himself to me if he could have, got kidney cancer at 16 and I had to put him down. I know now that had I changed his food, I might have been able to reverse his disease in a relatively short period, so I am even more heartbroken that the lights came on too late.

I have debated whether these chapters belong in this book, but the more I research, the more I am learning about human health while I am discovering about our fur baby's health.

All the same, things that I have been writing about are impacting our pets. By doing this research on our fur babies, I am learning more cutting-edge research, which is very useful information for me, and most likely will also be useful for you.

And yes, I let my pets down, and I was responsible for their early deaths. I didn't know. And now that I do, I need to share what I am learning with you so that you can take a more proactive approach and not lose your beloved pets before their time. We need to be better informed so that our pets also have a long and vibrant, healthy, happy life.

PETS AND TOXINS

This information will impact almost all of us. We love our pets. 68% of U.S. households own a pet. 60% of them are dogs, and 47% of them are cats. And we are their animal guardians. They are not making choices for themselves; we make them for them. This information is invaluable.

As I research, this information is also filling in the blanks in my understanding of toxins and human health.

You may know some of these things. But if you don't, and you read these chapters, it might make a difference in the health of your pet so that they will live longer.

The FDA has, for decades, allowed pet food to violate federal law.

An estimated six million dogs and nearly six million cats will be diagnosed with cancer this year. The experts that I have been listening to and reading about believe that 90% of this is due to environment and lifestyle, and only 10% is genetic.[213]

Animals have been impacted by the change in our food products and our environment much faster than we humans have been. What we are feeding our pets, the store-bought food we buy, is disgusting in most instances. The toxins do damage much more quickly to their little bodies than they do to us. This also explains why children exposed to GMOs, and other toxins, have a much higher rate of disease and illness now. Their little bodies cannot process the toxins out of their systems.

Epigenetics is an emerging field. I understand that experts believe you can either turn disease in your genes on or leave the light switch off. But I didn't understand the mechanism before reading how this works in animals. Metabolic damage from all these toxins causes defective genes. Not the other way around. There is some genetic connection to disease in animals caused by over breeding and a few other factors, but that only accounts for 10% of the diseases in animals. The balance is from the environment, which is mostly their food, and then also the other chemicals that are in their world, which includes dozens of unnecessary vaccines, topical pesticide applications, toxic cleaning supplies, and lawn chemicals like Glyphosate that are used where they run and play. Even the water we are giving them to drink has toxins in it if we haven't filtered it. The environment and lifestyle component include things like stress, sedentary lifestyle, toxins, pollution, infections, obesity, and of course, diet.

1 in 1.65 dogs will succumb to cancer.[214] And 1 in 3 cats. Your dog is four times more likely to get breast cancer than you are, eight times more likely to get bone cancer than you are, and up to 35 times more likely to get skin cancer than you are."[215] All these factors, over-vaccination, lawn chemicals, and food sprayed with chemicals are creating our pet's cancers. Also, the chemicals used for pest prevention on our pets are over-the-top toxic.

We have a reactive health care system for humans and our animals. We need to change to a proactive system if we want to heal our health, the health of our children, and the health of our pets. Reactive, in the current model, means our doctors go to school and learn how to identify symptoms of a disease, and then they learn from the pharmaceutical companies what drugs to use to treat those symptoms.[216] So, we're waiting until these animals get cancer, and then we have to talk about cutting it out, poisoning it out with chemotherapy, or burning it out with radiation.[217] Our doctors do not learn how to prevent cancer in the first place. Nor do they know how to stop other diseases that are escalating and more and more prevalent. Cancer is big business, so educating you as the animal guardian is the only solution.

What does that mean? You have read where I said in Chapter 23, "we are what we eat." If we are eating junk, then our bodies have no building blocks to build strong and healthy bodies. This is just as true for our animals as it is for us. We need to proactively find ways to feed our animals what Dr. Karen Becker, DMV calls "species-appropriate food."

How many humans hear that the drug prescribed for their ailment is the only solution to their health ills? Pet owners are also told that the only treatment available is to prescribe and utilize a pharmaceutical. Many owners are looking for a magic pill, just as they are for their own health. Changing diet is often not even considered, and when a knowledgeable Vet does recommend it, there is a lot of push back.

There is a small group of Holistic Vets that are proving that a change in diet can make an enormous difference in the health of your animal as I shared earlier in this book, food quality matters. When I share what we are feeding our pets, it's amazing that they survive even a few months, let alone a few years. It is disgusting. I am appalled.

Improve the quality of your animals' food, improve their health. (Improve the quality of your child's food, improve their health. Improve the quality of YOUR food, improve your health.)

Between the toxins and the bacteria that are in pet food, and the drugs that Vets are using, like steroids, to suppress the immune system, metabolic damage is rampant. Is this sounding familiar? It's the same problem with how conventional doctors are approaching our health.

Not only do Vets get little or no training in nutrition, they are heavily subsidized by pet food companies when they are in school. They receive free pet food every month to build brand loyalty, and pet food companies teach them it would be negligent to feed an animal anything but a balanced diet of pet food. These pet foods have nothing to do with what is species-appropriate food. Connecting the dots, I now eat the Paleo diet, and my health is improved because I am eating what my ancestors ate. I am now eating "species-specific" food. We need to feed our animals what is appropriate for them. This will vary by species, but it is not a high carbohydrate kibble. What is a high carbohydrate kibble? It is something that turns to pure sugar in the animal's system. And what feeds cancer? You got it, sugar.

Even young pups are getting cancer tumors. Just like our human babies are being born with over 250 chemicals right from the umbilical cord, newborn puppies and kitties are also being born with a heavy toxic load right at the beginning.

A dog or a cat in nature is hunting live food. It was interesting to read about all of this. I had an ah-ha moment when my doctor suggested that I eat pastured meat and organic vegetables and fruit. It made total sense to me. It resonated. It was like that I could have had a V-8 moment. Now that I know, I am learning what is appropriate for our pets in their wild state. Animals aren't even eating all the muscle of their kill, they are eating the intestine, which gives them the right probiotics and the undigested greens, and they are eating the organs. They leave the rest of the animal behind for the scavengers. (This certainly makes Dr. Terry Wahl's Protocol make more sense. She has helped thousands with multiple sclerosis (M.S.) by recommending a diet heavy on organ meat as well as fruits and vegetables.)

When I start to share with you what we are feeding our animals when we feed them store-bought animal food, it will gross you out. Or, at least it grossed me out. It's disgusting. And it couldn't be further away from what they would eat in the wild, starting with the word "fresh." Remember that word.

How did this happen? It has happened for the same reason that we are eating processed and fast food with synthetic chemicals and little food value. It has happened because of convenience. And it is far worse than the SAD (Standard American Diet) that Americans are eating. So, good grief, how do our animals live on this garbage diet as long they do?

Add to that, our pets are getting a double whammy from Glyphosate, Glyphosate (Roundup) is used on the GMO's in their food, and it is sprayed on the lawns they are enjoying outdoors. Our pets can't avoid these toxic chemicals.

Monsanto just recently lost three lawsuits concerning Glyphosate because the opposing attorneys forced Monsanto to release records during discovery that showed they knew these chemicals were causing cancer 20 years ago. Monsanto choose not to tell us until they had no choice.

The World Health Organization calls Roundup a probable carcinogen for humans. However, for animals, they say, is it a **known** carcinogen. And yet, this herbicide is still being sprayed on our crops. There are now 40,000 pending lawsuits against Monsanto for human illnesses. And yet, the EPA, just this week (2/20), declared there is no proof that Glyphosate is causing any human damage, cancer, or disease. My goodness, how much money is changing hands for the EPA to come to such an outrageous, ridiculous conclusion.

If you want to understand the whole controversy about Glyphosate, you can educate yourself by reading my chapters on food in my first book. I am not a scientist, but I voted with caution and eliminated as much of this herbicide as possible from my diet and my environment. It just didn't make sense to me that I should be eating toxins or "…cides." I recommend that you do the same. And since the landmark lawsuit in 2018 got the discovery from Monsanto that they had been deceiving us about the safety of their product and that Glyphosate is a carcinogen, it is outrageous that the EPA is declaring that there is no damage from these chemicals to the human body. There is damage to our bodies, to our animals, to our groundwater, and everywhere that our water runs off and as a result, it is killing our freshwater, lakes, oceans, and sea life. Furthermore, it is chelating all the minerals we need for a healthy body function right out of our dirt as we grow our plants and right out of our bodies as we eat items sprayed with the herbicide. And even worse, these chemicals are making us sick, our children sick and our pets sick.

I am going to divide this part of the book into five sections. What is in the food that we are feeding most of our animals (Chapter 27)? What should we be feeding our animals (Chapter 28)? I will give you resources so that you can sort out the best selections for your pet based on your budget; then, a chapter on vaccines (29) and another on steroids (30). As controversial as this subject is for our children, it is just as controversial for our animals and will explain the stranglehold that pharmaceutical companies have on our government, our conventional M.D.s, and our Vets. I won't make a recommendation since once again, I am not a doctor, but I sure as heck want to explain the problem as I understand it. Finally, I want to list plants that are dangerous to animals, so keep them away from your pets in the house, and essential oils and fragrances, and what I can find about their effect on our pets. I will share references where you can discover more on your own. This information is critical to you as a guardian of another living being (Chapter 31).

Just remember "…cides" means it kills something. That means "…cides" are killing us; they are killing our pets; they are killing our children. GMO's have toxins from different organisms spliced into them. Stay away. Don't believe our government telling us that they are just fine. Too much money, honey. Do like I have done, vote with caution. Even if they weren't harmful, ensuring that you aren't eating them just in case is prudent.

The most interesting quote I found is that 90% of oncologists would not take the same treatment on themselves for most cancers that they are administering to their patients, no matter whether it is an animal or a human. Think about that. Do your own research before you move forward and have a robust conversation with your oncologist. The treatment may indeed be the best option but know what you are accepting before you agree. Be a partner in the decision.

I also learned that Monsanto serves organic food in its cafeteria. Think about that.

And then continue reading my next chapter, but don't read it after a heavy meal.

Chapter 27

What the Heck Is in Your Purchased Pet Food? The Food Dilemma

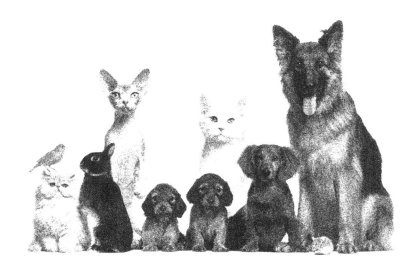

THE BIG TAKEAWAYS ON WHAT THE HECK IS IN YOUR PURCHASED PET FOOD? THE FOOD DILEMMA:[218]

- *Our pets are getting all the same diseases that humans are getting.*

- *They, too, are dealing with all the toxins, in and on their food, and in and on the ground that they go outside to romp on, and from what we are using for flea and tick control. They are also getting sick from the topicals we are using on their skin, as well as the vaccines that we are overloading their little bodies with as we over-vaccinate them.*

- *Some of this is mandated by our government, who support the pharmaceutical companies, even if the Vet believes something is causing the pet harm.*

- *Animals have faster metabolisms and age more quickly than humans. As a result, the lifestyle choices we make on their behalf "show up" much more quickly than they do in people.*

- *What do animals do in the wild? They hunt and eat their kill. They eat the fresh kill starting with the gut and the organs.*

- *We need to feed our pet companions species-specific food.*

- *Our kibble and our wet food for our pets start with what is known in the industry as the 4 Ds. It is made from animals that are*
  - *Disabled*
  - *Dead*
  - *Diseased*
  - *Dying*
- *This is hardly fresh food.*

- *These ingredients come at a bargain price, and pet food companies are buying them. Companies are making a profit selling restaurant waste, including rancid oils, ranch waste, packing house waste, chicken feathers, feet, and beak waste. It comes from roadkill and dead animals in the field that got thrown in the back of a truck and sat there and rotted until it could get to the rendering plant.*

- *It is not even remotely "species-specific" food. By its very nature, it is obvious that it is not good for your pet.*

"Gardening Rule-The richer your environment, the more resistant your plants are to disease."

DR. RICH PALMQUIST DVM THE TRUTH ABOUT PET CANCER

2018 This also applies to the human or animal gut biome

From the time I was born, I was madly in love with animals. At 3, I was running all over the neighborhood to pet the neighbor's pets. I had popped out very allergic to animals, but I didn't care, and even at 2½ or 3, I was very independent, and nothing would stop me. There was a heart connection with animals right from the beginning, and rashes were certainly not going to stop me.

One of my earliest memories is sitting on the door stoop of our next-door neighbor in Pennsylvania; I sat there with Penny, her dog. I had tons of allergies to food from the beginning as well, so Mrs. Schulich would buy oyster crackers for me (egg-free), and I would sit there and share them with Penny. One for me, one for Penny. I adored that little dog. (And still have vivid memories of this.)

My parents finally broke down sometime after this and adopted a puppy. A big dog in the neighborhood attacked it, and the pup died. Even at this early age (under 4), the heartbreak was overwhelming. And memorable. I can see the living room in my mind's eye, where we all sat to mourn the loss of this poor little being.

As I grew, I became an avid reader, and quickly learned that I couldn't read famous books about animals. They were too painful. Books like **Big Yeller**, **Black Beauty**, **My Friend Flicka**, and **The Yearling** created a terrible pain in my heart, so I started to avoid anything that would create that experience for me.

We got another dog when I was 7, and Heidi, a dachshund, lived until I was in my 20's. She was my best friend and companion.

We had a postman who kicked the next-door neighbor's Cocker Spaniel, Rosie, and the dog snipped and bit him, just a little, but it did break the skin. I was furious with the mailman, who wanted the dog put down. I saw what happened and stood up for this sweet dog, and the postman finally stood down. I was maybe 8.

I have had pets for much of my life. When I got married the first time, we got cats, and for the rest of my adult life, I have had multiple cats and adore them as much as I adore dogs. I love all animals.

I wanted to share these memories so that you understand a little bit about why it is so important for me to share what I am writing about today.

As you know, when I got an autoimmune disease, and my doctor was clueless about what was wrong with me, I started my research to discover what was making me sick and causing my body to hurt. For the six years that I researched, I never connected the dots, that the same things I was discovering about my health, the same environmental toxins, the same issues with our food supply, were also issues for my cats.

My friends used to tease me that in their next life, they wanted to come back as my cat. Ha! But now that I am researching what is happening with our fur babies, I am learning that I did a terrible job as the guardian for my last kitties. Everything had changed, but I missed it. And, as a result, my heart is broken once again, and I feel that it is necessary that I share all this information with you.

I didn't know. I should have figured it out, but I was so focused on my health, I did not focus on my pets. My cats always lived good healthy lives well into their 20's. These cats died at 12, 14, and 16, and they all died of cancer. What has impacted me the most is that it didn't have to happen. Even as my last little red hair boy Beeper got sick, had I changed his food, I have learned that I may have been able to save him.

All this information started to become public two years ago, but with all my research on health, I should have figured it out.

I just learned that the average age for a domestic cat now is 12, but that this doesn't have to be. Our pets should live well into their 20's like my previous kitties did. ***Dogs should too, and their average age now is 10.*** I just watched a video of a "dawg" that was 36, and healthy and happy.

The early demise of my kitties has haunted me. The only thing that I could figure out was that GMOs entered the food stream in 1996 and were in full use by 1998. Cat food had changed from previous pet food. So, I figured out that this was the place to start to research about pets. I am sad to share; it's far worse than my wildest dreams.

Our pets are getting the same diseases that humans are getting. And they too, are dealing with all the toxins, in and on their food, and in and on the ground that they go outside to romp on, from what we are using for flea control. They are also getting sick from the topicals we are using on their skin, as well as the vaccines that we are overloading their little bodies with as we over-vaccinate them. And some of this is mandated by our government, who support the pharmaceutical companies. Even if the Vet believes something is causing the pet harm, he is forced to comply.

It's been great to do this research because I am learning things about human health from the Holistic Vets that I am reading and listening to as they explain the problems they are encountering, and some of their comments are filling in the dots about human health. I am learning more about our children's health at the same time. What children have in common with animals is smaller body size. Their little bodies can't deal with the number of toxins they are encountering. Their bodies don't stand a chance to process them out. Toxins accumulate in children's bodies. By the time a child is 5, he has eaten 7 pounds of toxins.[219] With animals, it becomes even more complicated, because their metabolism is faster, so the toxins impact their little bodies even harder.

"Animals have faster metabolisms and age more quickly than humans. As a result, the lifestyle choices we make on their behalf 'show up' much more quickly than they do in people."

THE TRUTH ABOUT PET CANCER[220]

As a pet guardian, you control what you feed your pet and what your pet gets to drink. You control how much exercise your animal gets, and the kind of medical attention they receive throughout their life. Your furry baby relies upon you to make decisions for them on their behalf. As a pet parent, you choose what quality of life you create for your pet, so choose wisely.

Some of what I want to share with you will be the same message that you read about earlier in this book when I was discussing our food habits and how to care for our children. I guess it should not be a surprise that it's the same thing for our animals. And if you didn't want to hear it for your health, hopefully, you will pay attention when I discuss this regarding your pets.

Often when I speak, someone approaches me and states, "your information is all fine and well, but it has nothing to do with me." They point out that I am not speaking to their pain point. (my words) They are healthy, so they have no intention of cleaning up the toxins and, therefore, being "deprived." I should put DEPRIVED in caps. It is such a huge objection.

I was very frustrated by this in the beginning, and a wise friend told me it was my job to share the information, but that I was not responsible for what people did with the information. I was the messenger, but the people listening were responsible for how they used the information. My challenge is to reframe my message so that more and more people will "hear" it.

Research shows that it can take as many as 17 hits before someone starts to "hear" the information and use it to change. I get it.

But somehow, I feel that many of our relationships with our animals are so heart-connected and that we will hear the message faster when I explain that animals do not have a choice. They live with what we feed them. They live with what is in their environment. We are their caretakers, and we owe it to them to grant them the best life possible.

I am not suggesting that a Mother doesn't want to protect her children, but the problem is what I talk about is not mainstream. Everyone else is eating the SAD, the Standard American Diet. And the bonus for them is that the SAD is so friggin convenient. So even though it's about their children, who they love more than life, they don't "hear" the message. Everyone else is eating processed and fast foods too. Why shouldn't they eat this food?

So, let me go back to the basics, but this time regarding pets.

- Food Quality Matters
- Food is Information
- Food Heals
- Processed Food and Fast Food have little nutritional value. They have ingredients that you don't recognize, and your body or the pet's body doesn't recognize them either. Pet food is overly processed.
- Our System is Reactive, not Proactive.
- When our animals get sick, we take them to the Vet. When we get sick, we go to a conventional MD. Our MDs and DMVs are trained to match a pill to the ailment. Their main source of information is their pharmaceutical rep. This is reactive. We have all been responding after the illness is evident.
- Glyphosate is toxic to our bodies. It chelates the minerals out of our soil and then doesn't allow us to absorb what minerals we do get into our gut.[221]
- Leaky gut is just as prevalent in our pets as it is in humans. What creates "Leaky Gut?" One of the causes is bad bacteria (Glyphosate is an antibiotic and kills all the good bacteria leaving the bad bacteria in our gut). Sensitivities, stress, parasites, and hormones also cause leaky gut. It is caused by toxins, which are everywhere in their world but especially in

their food, which is dead food. Toxins are also often on the public grasses where we are walking our pets.

- What is the purpose of bad bacteria in our gut, and why don't we want it? Bad bacteria are there to begin the decomposition process (death).[222] Yuk. Whether or not it's for your gut or your animal's gut, foster healthy good bacteria.
- The body wants to heal, but it needs strong building blocks for that to happen. Cells in our bodies are constantly being replaced, and we need healthy building blocks to do that.
- BPA, a lining of cans and BHP, a preservative put into pet food, are both Endocrine Disruptors for our animals and our bodies.
- Inherited DNA is not always the cause of disease. Instead, 90% of the time, the diseases we inherited in our DNA **are activated** by damage to the Mitochondria. We can turn the switch on or off by what we eat and what is in our environment.
- Processed Food and Fast Food are Fake Industrial Foods. They are dead foods. They are toxic. There are very few nutrients in these "foods."
- Our conventional MD's hear a complaint and prescribe a pill. Our Vets are doing the same thing, and even worse, we are expecting the pill or the shot to cure the ills of our pets. We WANT a magic pill.
- Conventional MD's and Vets receive little or no education in school about nutrition and don't understand the importance of nutrition. We keep expecting a magic pill to heal us, and the MD or Vet accommodates us by prescribing a pill. But it is NOT magic and doesn't cure the ill.
- Our Doctors and our Vets are not taught that food is information. And, they do not learn that food impacts our health or our pets' health.
- We are resistant to change when it comes to the food in our diet and the food in our pets' diet.
- Vets are taught that the animal must eat food, that is:
    - Over processed
    - Balanced
    - Manufactured by the pet food industry
- Vets are given free pet food monthly to build brand loyalty to this "dead" food.

Because animal food is over-processed, it has no real food value. Our animal food is composed of chemicals stuck together with sugar. Synthetic vitamins are added, which the animal's body often cannot use.[223] Most synthetic vitamins have not been tested or monitored for safety.

- Scraps from the table will UNBALANCE the diet of the pet and should not be allowed. **This will harm your pet.** (I have a solution to this in Chapter 28.)
- People take their pets to the Vet and are looking for the magic pill. Changing the animal's diet is often their last resort, and there is often great resistance. But often this is the one thing that finally makes a difference in our pets' health.
- We are opting for convenience for our bodies, our families, and our pets. We are not opting for real food that will supply the nutrients that our bodies and our animal's bodies need to survive and be vibrant.
- Just as I discovered when researching for my first book, companies run their own studies and monitor their products for safety. ***Profits win over health every time.***
- The #1 objection to buying and feeding our loved ones an organic diet is budgetary. But we spend much more in the long run if we add in the health care costs down the line.

Let's stop for a moment and discuss—what do animals do in the wild? They hunt and eat their kill. They eat the fresh kill starting with the gut and the organs. The gut offers them nice beautiful probiotics and beautiful chlorophyll. The organs are very mineral-rich. This is their species-appropriate diet. Their bodies can handle the bacteria from their kill. Their digestive s system is designed so that they have very short digestive tracks to move bacteria out of their bodies quickly. The only difference between cats and dogs is that cats are completely carnivorous, and dogs are carnivorous but do eat some plants. Cats will never stop and eat an already dead animal. They catch and kill their food and eat it fresh. And by the way, cats do not eat fish in nature. (This was a surprise for me, I fed my kitties so much canned fish).

Bells and whistles went off with this. Terry Wahl, an MD who has MS, was bedridden and told she didn't have long to live. She had two small children, so she started her research because she refused to accept that there was nothing medicine could do to help her heal. The bottom line is that she figured out how to bring herself back to wellness. Her protocol has now been used to help thousands of others return to relative wellness. What is different about her recommended diet? It is heavily weighed on eating organ meat from pastured animals and then eating organic fruits and vegetables. Fully functional once again, she now teaches at the University of Iowa, and she rides her bike several miles round trip to work each day.

After getting sick, I now eat Paleo, which is a species-specific food for me. Paleo is how my ancestors, the cavemen, ate. I am working towards eating Pegan, which is mostly organic fruits and vegetables with small amounts of pastured meats (the size of the palm of my hand.) Vegan would also be species-specific food for humans.

Neither humans nor animals are foraging for dead, processed food that contains chemicals and fake vitamins. They aren't looking for simple carbohydrates; they aren't looking for sugar. And they aren't in the wild searching for cans or pellets with chemicals and preservatives or fake supplements.

These factors are the complete antithesis of their "species-specific diet."

Let's look at what is in manufactured "balanced" animal food, both wet and kibble. This food is the stuff that Vets learned in Veterinary School is the only food that is healthy for you to feed your animal. The truth is quite the opposite.

And, let's look at where pet food comes from, and what is in it, and then why it is harming our pets.

Our kibble and our wet food for our pets start with what is known in the industry as the 4 Ds. It is made from animals that are:

- Disabled
- Dead

- Diseased
- Dying

This is hardly fresh food.

These ingredients come at a bargain price, and pet food companies are buying them. Companies are making a profit selling restaurant waste, including rancid oils, ranch waste, packing house waste, chicken feathers, feet, and beak waste. It comes from roadkill and dead animals in the field that got thrown in the back of a truck and sat there and rotted until it could get to the rendering plant.

It is not even remotely "species-specific" food. And by its very nature, it is obvious that it is not good for your pet.

I am discussing most commercially available pet food. If you are making homemade animal food, there are also pitfalls that I will discuss later in this section. But if you are buying anything off the shelf, my comments are valid, and you may need to rethink what you are feeding your animal.

Let's start with this.

"The FDA has, for decades, allowed pet food to violate federal law. The FDA allows diseased animal tissue and dead animal carcasses (non-slaughtered) to be processed into pet food even though this material is a direct violation of federal law, with no disclosure to the consumer which pet foods contain this (and other) illegal, risky material."[224] The Association for Truth in Pet Food has had a petition with the FDA since 2016 and just got this response in January 2020:

Enforcing pet food law "would not be in the public interest."

Huh? What in the world is our government thinking?

The EPA, another government agency recently declared there is no human health threat from Glyphosate. This statement came after three lawsuits against Monsanto were won, showing that Glyphosate causes human cancer and after Monsanto released records in discovery in the lawsuit that showed Monsanto had known for 20 years that their product caused cancer. The lawsuit was won in 2018, and the EPA just made this conclusion in January 2020. What??? There are now 40,000 lawsuits pending against Monsanto.

Our government is not going to protect us. Whether it is the FDA regarding pet food or the EPA regarding toxic chemicals being sprayed on our food, they are NOT protecting us. Who are they protecting, in my opinion? Big business interests, no matter how dangerous that support is for us, the public. Our government has failed us, and they are also failing our pets. YOU MUST DO YOUR RESEARCH AND PROTECT YOURSELF AND YOUR LOVED ONES.

Our kibble and our wet food for our pets come from waste, disgusting waste.

The rendering process develops chemicals that are deadly and cause cancer. It is far from optimal nutrition. And it most certainly is not "balanced" for the pet to eat.

When you take proteins and caramelize them, the chemical compounds that this creates cause cancer. Your average dog eats 122 times more advanced chemicals from this caramelization process than humans eat, and a cat eats 38 times more. We are feeding them cancer-causing chemicals that are created in these tubs.[225]

Another chemical that is produced by cooking this conglomeration at high heat is acrylamide, which is also a known carcinogen.

The common word for these ingredients on labels is "by-products."

This toxic goo is then added to either grain or legumes, peas, potatoes, and tapioca. The grains are drenched in Roundup (Glyphosate), a carcinogen; the legumes, peas, potatoes, etc. are GMOs that have BT Toxin in them. I understand from the Institute of Responsible Technology that BT Toxin is also poison and creates allergies in our bodies and our animals' bodies. Roundup doesn't allow minerals from the ground to travel to our gut. BT toxin doesn't allow the minerals that made it into the animal's gut to be absorbed. The minerals get chelated right back out. And then synthetic vitamins and food dyes get added to this goo. Mind you, food dyes cause behavioral problems, and the animals are color blind, so this is purely for the owners. Preservatives get added, also chemicals, and to top it off, *carrageenan* is added, which destroys the gut wall even more. *Carrageenan* is a known carcinogen.

For this disgusting mixture to become kibble, it must be 40% - 50% sugar. The carbs (Grains, legumes, peas, potatoes, tapioca) turn into sugar. And what feeds cancer? You got it, sugar.[226] Sugar also does damage to every organ in our body and our pet's body.

This toxic combination damages the mitochondria, which then turns the tendency towards cancer in the genes on. Animals are not getting cancer because they inherited genes to get cancer; they are getting cancer because the switch is turned on that causes cancer. And then the sugar feeds cancer. It's a vicious cycle.

The best thing to say about all of this is that it is cheap. The animal will eat it because it's the food he has been fed. He can't say, hey; this is not good food for me. And although I have not read this, I am betting that that animal becomes addicted to the sugar, so he overeats and gains weight, which is a whole new problem for animal health. This is how sugar impacts we humans, so it makes sense that it also impacts our pets this way. Sugar is eight times more addictive than heroin, so it probably is addictive to our animals as well. This causes weight gain, another animal health issue that shortens their life.

None of this has anything to do with species-specific food, which is what we all need to survive. Wild wolves and cats don't go running around looking for carbohydrates or sugar. They don't look for preservatives. And they don't look for rendered goo.

Here's the thing, I read more than one account that an owner with a sick pet at the Vet resists when the Vet suggests that they change the animal's food. People do NOT understand that food is medicine both for their animal's body and for theirs. They are still in reactive mode. Give my animal a pill, give my pet a shot, keep them overnight, and let's go from there, yadda de yadda.

But then, **when the pet owner finally agrees to change the food, health happens.** There have been instances where the health of the animal improved in a matter of weeks. Once the mindset goes from reactive to proactive, their health changes for the better, it's a miracle, or is it? Read below why changing the diet to a healthier biologically appropriate diet can be the miracle that pet owners are looking for.

I am far from the first person to become appalled by what is actually in animal food. Many Pet owners have done their research, and they do want to feed their animals nutritious food. They don't want to feed their pets dead food or rendered food and are demanding better.

But what this has done is open the power of marketing. What manufacturers say about their pet food is not regulated. Owners read the labels but don't know what the ingredients are. The deception is remarkable. Words like "premium" are bogus. Even "organic" on a pet food label is not regulated.

"For the record, neither clean eating nor clean labels have an official definition, however, generally speaking, eating clean "… is about eating whole foods, or 'real' foods—those that are unprocessed or minimally processed, refined, and handled, making them as close to their natural form as possible." According to Go Clean Label:

> *Clean label is a consumer-driven movement, demanding a return to 'real food' and transparency through authenticity. Food products containing natural, familiar, simple ingredients that are easy to recognize, understand, and pronounce. No artificial ingredients or synthetic chemicals.*[227]

KAREN BECKER, DVM WHO IS AN EXPERT ON HOLISTIC PET FOOD AND PART OF THE MERCOLA GROUP.

It is virtually impossible to make rendered food anything remotely like real whole food that is nutritious, so it has all been marketing hype to meet the consumer demand. Pet food companies see the opportunity to sell healthier food but are using it to deceive us with new wording. Products that they are delivering to store shelves are as far away from species-specific as they were before.

> *"The pet food industry is no different than leading food marketers for humans when it comes to cheap substitutes and false health claims," says the report's lead author, Linley Dixon, Ph.D., a policy analyst at The Cornucopia Institute,[228] an organic watchdog organization.*

"An ever-growing number of pet parents have become too knowledgeable about pet nutrition to keep buying big pet food's products. The industry continues to ignore the need to explore connections between an exploding number of pets with degenerative diseases, and continue the practice of feeding dogs and cats a biologically inappropriate processed diet day in and day out for months, years, or a lifetime."[229]

Beware of pet food with rice as an ingredient. The Truth about Pet Food has found very high levels of arsenic in pet foods with rice. *"Even though the legal safety limit of total iAs content might not be surpassed in most pet foods, iAs is considered a non-threshold carcinogen, and any exposure constitutes a health risk."[230] "In human beings, chronic exposure to iAs has been associated with tumors of the skin, bladder, and lungs, and with alterations in gastrointestinal, neurological, cardiovascular, immunological, hematological, pulmonary, and developmental function. In dogs, research has mainly focused on nephrotoxicity* (toxicity in the kidneys)."

The Cornucopia report is accusing the pet food industry of knowingly using inferior products, carcinogens, cheap ingredients, and harmful preservatives in our animal products, placing profits beyond what should be acceptable for what they are selling for animal food.

The Cornucopia Report agrees with findings by the Truth about Pet Cancer group and the Institute for Responsible Technology and points out the practices of the major pet food companies to coverup the products that are causing harm to our pets.

Although products that state "certified organic" on the label are generally a better choice, because of lack of regulation, that is not always true. They still might include dangerous and unnecessary ingredients.

Furthermore, The Truth About Pet Food has been trying to get definitions from the FDA about what is allowed under ingredients on pet food labels. As a matter of fact, pet food ingredient definitions are very different than the human food counterparts; pet owners are denied public access to ANY pet food ingredient definitions by the FDA. The FDA has an agreement with AAFCO. This was their response: the FDA said "*no*"—pet owners will not be allowed to know what is in their pet's food because it is "confidential commercial information." The FDA MUST know what they are. They are entrusted with enforcing them.

This is ridiculous. We should not accept this. This is another reason why buying quality food and making your pet food is crucial. We need to vote with our dollars here as well.

"FDA testing has found sodium pentobarbital, the drug used to euthanize animals, in at least 30 different pet foods."

This report is accusing pet food manufacturers of including the carcasses of companion animals in the mix. Pet food companies deny this and say the proof is that there is no DNA detectable in pet food from companion animals, but the truth is that once it goes into the rendering pot, all DNA is no longer detectable because it has gone under intense heat.

"High prices do not necessarily imply high quality. Illusive labels and deceptive marketing are used by many companies to disguise substandard food."[231]

These pet foods consist of large amounts of grains, like corn, wheat, rice and oats, and peas and potatoes, which are not species-appropriate for the animal and which are either sprayed with Roundup or are GMOs, which added additional toxins to the animal's diet. In addition, Cornucopia recommends avoiding labels with these grains because the grains used are often moldy, offering dangerous mycotoxins into the mix.

Carrageenan is then added as well, along with BHA, BHT Propyl Gallate, and ethoxyquin all toxic ingredients.

> "When looking at pet food labels, look for natural antioxidants such as tocopherols, vitamin C, and flavonoids. These are a better choice over synthetic preservatives."[232]

Animal studies have repeatedly shown that food-grade carrageenan causes gastrointestinal inflammation and cancer at lower doses than the average daily intake. Given the high rates of colon cancer in both dogs and cats, I highly recommend removing carrageenan from your pet's diet.

DR. MICHAEL DYM, DVM.

I also found a reference connecting carrageenan to colon cancer in human health.[233]

And it is not a surprise that carrageenan manufacturers are working overtime to discredit all of the research that their products are harmful. (Again, check your labels, carrageenan is in many, many of our human products from milk, to cosmetics to toothpaste).

The effects of ill health on our animals is exacerbated by the fact that animals eat the same food every day. As humans, at least we get to vary our diets. The cumulative exposure is what is one of the things causing disease in our pets more quickly than exposure to us humans.

Even though claims that the food is GMO-Free on labels, Cornucopia writes that the only way to ensure that the animals that went into the pet food mix were not fed GMOs is to buy certified organic food. The government has no laws to enforce whether the food is GMO-free or not. Manufacturers have gone so far as to include new round insignias, that fool the eye that they are non-GMO or organic, but which are instead, meaningless.

Regulatory rules protect the pet food manufacturers, not the consumer. Good grief.

Beyond the obvious, I want to address why all of this is so important to your pet's health.

I explained in my first book, **It Feels Good to Feel Good, Learn to Eliminate Toxins, Reduce Inflammation and Feel Great Again,** what happens in the human gut when it gets a diet of processed and fast food. We get a "leaky gut." Leaky gut is important to understand in order for us to heal our gut and return to relative health. It is through our gut that we absorb all our nutrients, and by giving our bodies the correct building blocks, it can heal us because we are absorbing these beautiful nutrients.

It's exactly the same thing in our pets. The gut wall becomes destroyed by similar issues when we feed our pet's food that is not biologically correct or species-specific for our pet. A high carbohydrate diet becomes sugar in the gut and causes leaks in the gut wall. Parasites, toxins, chemicals (there are over 70,000 chemicals in our lives now), infections, medications including antibiotics, over vaccinations, sensitivities, stress all cause leaks in our pets' gut walls. When the animals' gut gets "leaky," the pets' immune system begins to attack itself just like our immune system does from the same things. The gut is the key to the animal's health.

"The more food is processed, the more nutrient-depleted and chemically altered it becomes. In order to compensate for the loss of taste, various chemicals are added during processing, including flavor enhancers, colors, various additives, and preservatives. By negatively altering the gut flora, processed foods play an important part in damaging the intestinal tract. It is increasingly clear that dietary influences on the intestinal flora are involved in health and disease.[234]

The gut lining in humans is only one cell thick. It is thinner than a piece of tissue paper. It heals itself every seven days, but eventually, it can't keep up if it is being bombarded by all the negative things listed above. I didn't find any information on dog's or cat's animal gut lining, but it is logical that it also would be very thin. The way this mechanism works is that the gut lining must be thin so that nutrients that nourish both our bodies (our pets and our human bodies) can pass into the bloodstream. It's the nutrients that we want to pass through, and these nutrients need to be strong building blocks so that the body can do all its important processes.

To help your pet heal, it all begins with the quality of the food you are feeding your pet. I list places you can go to find better food in Chapter 28 but understanding why "species-specific" food is the solution to healing your pet's gut will help them return to health. This explains the "why" this is so important.

It's also important to eliminate other chemicals in your dog and cat's life. The same environmental chemicals that are harmful to our bodies are harmful to our pet's bodies. I list all the places where I found chemicals in my first book, and I share what I found to replace them that were lower toxin. This is important for you to utilize in order to be able to lower your toxic load, and for you to lower your pet's toxic load.

If you want a healthy body, if you want your children to have a healthy body and if you want your pet to be healthy, lower the toxic load from their food and from their environment.

Start with quality food for your pet. Species-specific food is the most important thing you can do for your pet's health.

I had a cat that was throwing up and getting diarrhea all the time. I could have helped her if I had changed her diet. I would take her to the Vet and get her a shot. Had I changed her food; she would have lived a healthier life. She was also overweight, 20 pounds, which was because of the carbohydrate quantity in her food. Had I changed her diet; she would have returned to a more appropriate weight. I didn't know how to help her, and neither did my Vet. Making these changes to her food was never suggested.

All 3 of my kitties got cancer. Had I changed their food to a species-specific food, I could have avoided them getting cancer, and probably helped them return to health.

I did change my diet to eating for nutrients, and that changed my health. You need to do the same for your pets.

The gut is key to your animal's health, and the way to heal the gut is to feed our animals the correct diet. It's the key to keeping your animal disease-free, and if they are showing signs of ill health, it's the key to returning your fur baby back to good health.

Just a note, most conventional MD's are not identifying "leaky gut" as the root cause of illness. This is something that has been studied and addressed by the functional medicine group of doctors who practice "root cause" medicine. I am a big believer in the functional medicine approach because it saved my life. They are real MDs that went for additional training because most of them got sick, and they couldn't help themselves. Addressing "leaky gut" is something you can do for yourself without your MD, so it's important that you are aware of it and pay attention to it.

Similarly, most Vets will not know about "Leaky Gut" nor will they address it. They didn't learn about it in Veterinary School, which is heavily influenced by the pharmaceutical industry and the pet food industry. You would need to go to a Holistic Vet to work with a Vet that understands how this mechanism works in your pet's body. Again, this is something that you can start to address on your own to improve your pet's health.

In other words, find the right doctors to support your health and the health of your pet. Changing your food is a great beginning. Start by changing the things you control in your own life and your animal's life. Then, the right doctor can help you address the other things that are disrupting your health and your animal's health.

In my next chapter, we are going to discuss possible solutions to this dead, rendered, dubious, and processed crud that we have been feeding our pets. There are different possibilities to meet each person's budget. But please, look at the highest level of food that you can afford for your pet. Your pet's life depends on it.

Additional sources to understand the gut health of your pet:

> https://feline-nutrition.org/health/feline-inflammatory-bowel-disease-nature-and-treatment
> https://blog.paleohacks.com/signs-your-dog-has-leaky-gut/#
> https://simplewag.com/leaky-gut-syndrome-in-dogs/

Chapter 28

What should I feed my pet?

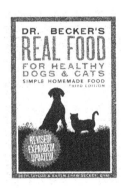

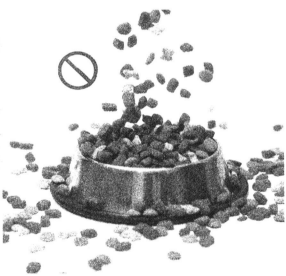

THE BIG TAKEAWAYS ON WHAT SHOULD I FEED MY PET?[235]

> - *Our pets are getting all the same diseases that humans are getting.*
>
> - *Dr. Karen Becker recommends that you feed your pet the best food that you can afford. If you cannot afford top quality food, then feed the pet a couple of high-quality meals a week. If that is impossible, feed your pet high-quality snacks. Some high-quality food is better than none.*
>
> - *Homemade food either can be the best thing you serve your animal, or it can be the most dangerous thing you serve your animal. It all depends on whether you do a careful formulation with nutrients that make it balanced.*
>
> - *Dr. Becker has a cookbook on Amazon with recipes that will ensure your animals' health if you choose to cook for your pet.*
>
> - *You can't forget that animal food made with grains or legumes, corn, potatoes, and tapioca are all loaded with Glyphosate and/ or BT Toxin (GMO's). They are poisons. Organic is the only way to avoid these ingredients. Grains may also have mycotoxins from mold.*
>
> - *You need to feed your pet some species-specific food and avoid some over the counter animal foods. See your options below. Use the highest level you can afford for your pet.*

So, now that we are aware of the deception and all the misleading practices, what do we do to protect our animals and feed them healthy food?

Cornucopia's first recommendation is to buy pet food that is certified organic. Next, they recommend that you consider making your pet food from quality ingredients. If you choose this option, you must follow a recipe and make sure that the food truly is balanced.

How do you know what to do? There are several lists now that expose the best and the worst foods on the market.

These are Dr. Karen Becker's recommendations on how to feed your pets. Dr. Becker is a Vet associated with Dr. Mercola, a holistic health care professional.

Feed Your Pet the Best Diet You Can Reasonably Afford[236]

What pet guardians need to keep in mind is that whatever they feed their pet, it should be high moisture, high protein, moderate fat, and low carb to be healthy for your animal. Next, it needs to be nutritionally balanced, which I will comment on below.

Her recommendation is to not think in terms of all or nothing. If you can feed your animal, an organic home-cooked balanced meal every day, great, but if not think in terms of a couple of days of home-cooked balanced food, and if you can't do that, think in terms of homemade treats to supplement what you are feeding your pet. Studies have shown that some healthy food is better than no healthy food at all.

Homemade food can be either the best food you serve your animal, or it can be the most dangerous thing you serve your animal. It needs to be a high-quality formulation with the correct nutrients that makes it balanced. Dr. Becker's cookbook explains how to do that for the optimal health of your pet.

You can't forget that animal food with grains, legumes, corn, potatoes, and tapioca has Glyphosate and or BT Toxin. They are poisons. Organic is the only way to avoid these ingredients.

Following is Dr. Becker's list from Best to Worst:[237]

1. Nutritionally balanced raw homemade diet

    The good news about making your pet's food is you control the ingredients. You control the quality.

    The bad news is that it's not so easy to make balanced pet food, so you need to know what you are doing, or you could create harm to your pet even though you have the best of intentions.

    Homemade diets can fall far short in trace minerals, antioxidants including nutrients like manganese, magnesium, vitamin E and D, copper, zinc, iron, choline, and essential fatty acids.[238]

Since ethical practices in pet food are so difficult to trust, this is your best option if you make homemade food for your animal correctly. Dr. Becker has a cookbook for pet food available on Amazon if you want to choose this option. Her recipes provide you with ways to prepare perfectly balanced raw pet food. Dr. Becker also advises on the supplements that are important to add for balance.

She included supplements to add and in what quantities to make the food perfectly balanced.

2. "Nutritionally balanced cooked homemade diet—This option gives you all of the benefits of the homemade raw diet above, minus the benefits of the free enzymes and phytonutrients found in living foods. Interestingly, there are a few nutrients that are more bioavailable when cooked, for example, lycopene."[239]

Some animals prefer this. Some owners prefer this. Some medical conditions demand this.

Again, it is important to add the correct balance of supplements to make it healthy food for your pet.

3. Commercially available balanced raw food diet

This is the fastest-growing category available on the market. However, foods vary dramatically, and quality varies as well. If you choose this route, you MUST do your research.

Investigate the company you're buying from to make sure you're feeding the correct product for your pet's specific nutritional and medical goals. Read the original article from Dr. Becker noted in the endnotes to see all the factors you should take under consideration before you buy. You must learn to write, ask, confirm, and compare ingredients. Remember that what goes into the food one month could differ at another time, so keep asking and questioning.

4. A dehydrated or freeze-dried raw diet

    This is not quite the same as a balanced raw food diet, but it's stable to keep it on the shelf, and you just need to add water.

    "Dehydrated or freeze-dried raw diets haven't been processed at high temperatures. In many cases, the nutrient value has been retained minus a balanced fatty acid profile."[240]

    Make sure you choose a brand that is nutritionally balanced for all life phases.

5. Commercially available cooked or refrigerated food

    A fast-growing category of pet food. The food has been lightly cooked. The moisture content is excellent. The food is fresher than processed food and is a better choice than items lower on this list.

    You can find this food in refrigerated sections of pet food stores and some human grocery stores.

    Do your research, brands vary from terrible to quite nutritious, so make sure you know what you are buying. write, ask, confirm, and compare ingredients

6. Human-grade canned food

    Look up the package label on the manufacturer's website. If it doesn't say "human-grade," assume that it is not.

    These foods are much more expensive than feed grade or animal grade pet foods.

    You will most likely find these in animal boutique stores.

7. Super-premium canned food

    Found in Big Box stores and Vet Clinics. Better moisture than dry food. Not approved for human consumption. Quality varies. Some have excellent protein, fat, fiber, and carb ratios.

8. Human-grade dry food

    Loaded with carbohydrates. Not species-specific food. The ingredients have passed quality inspections and do not contain unidentified, rendered animal products.

    If the food was baked, it would note that on the label. Otherwise, it does have some carcinogenic ingredients.

9. Super-premium dry food

    Made from feed-grade ingredients and could harbor mycotoxins. The grain used not only had Glyphosate on it, but it was also likely moldy when it went into the food. High carbohydrate content. Not species-specific food. Available at big box retailers and some Veterinary clinics. Typically, naturally preserved.

10. Grocery store brand canned food

    Moisture content is better than Super-premium dry food, but these are loaded with harmful preservatives and grains, including butylated hydroxyanisole (BHA) and butylated hydroxytoluene (BHT), and ethoxyquin.

11. Grocery store brand dry food

    Same issues as 10 except low moisture

12. Semi-moist pouched food

    This category stunned me. When my Beeper stopped eating, I was handfeeding him these pouches. It hastened his demise.

"This stuff is really bad. The reason it is so far down the list is because in order to make the food semi-moist, the manufacturers must add an ingredient called propylene glycol. Propylene glycol is an undesirable preservative that is closely related to ethylene glycol, which is antifreeze. While propylene glycol is approved for use in pet foods, it's unhealthy for dogs and cats to consume."[241]

13. Unbalanced homemade diet, raw or cooked

This was also a surprise. Dead last on the list. I listened to several podcasts with Vets, and they talked about the danger of feeding your pet scraps, and now I understand why this is so deadly.

"Some pet owners believe they can offer their dog or cat a chicken breast and some veggies and call it a day. Many caring pet owners are unfortunately sorely lacking in knowledge about their companion animal's nutritional requirements.

Feeding fresh homemade food is a good thing; however, if the diet you're offering your pet is nutritionally unbalanced, it can cause significant, irreversible, and even potentially fatal health problems. These include endocrine abnormalities, skeletal issues, and organ degeneration as a result of deficiencies in calcium, trace minerals, and essential fatty acids."[242]

Almost every Veterinarian has seen animal patients that have been harmed by well-meaning owners who feed unbalanced diets. It's heartbreaking and entirely preventable. Homemade pet diets must be done right or not at all." [243]

If you want to make balanced homemade food for your pet, Dr. Becker has an animal cookbook available on Amazon. The link is below. I also found a cat food recipe that I share.

http://bit.ly/drBeckeranimalfoodrecipes
http://bit.ly/catfoodrecipe

Dr. Becker commented that you should buy the best food you can afford. Even serving healthy treats is valuable for your pet.

This is Dr. Morgan DMV's a Holistic Vet's pet treat recipe:

> http://bit.ly/healthyanimaltreatrecipe

Carrots and organic apples are also good treats. Do NOT feed your pet peanut butter.

Remember that variety is also important.

Lists of food that are rated for your pet. I found three that are very valuable from sources that I trust.

1. https://www.cornucopia.org/pet-food-guide/

    I also found this list on the Institute for Responsible Technology website

    1st: USDA Organic certified AND Non-GMO project verified.

    These pet foods offer the most rigorous testing and oversight to provide the healthiest option.

    2nd: USDA Organic.

    This certification provides food that has minimal GMO contaminants and free of synthetic fertilizers.

    3rd: Non-GMO Project Verified.

    This verification provides food that has been tested for minimal contamination of GMO ingredients.

    They have also compiled a list of recommended foods that you can purchase. You sign up for their mailing list, and it takes you directly to the list.

2. https://petsandgmos.com/best_for_pets/

    Their list included foods and treats that are not harmful to your pet.

The Truth about Pet Food, an advocacy group for better animal food and increased transparency, also has a list. They are doing great work and are requesting a donation that could be as small as $10 to get their list of approved pet foods.

3. http://www.truthaboutpetfoodstore.com/2020-list/

Let's talk about Leaky Gut and your pet for a moment. The things that cause Leaky Gut in humans are the same things that create Leaky Gut in our pets.

- Stress
- Toxins/ Chemicals/ GMO's/ Glyphosate (Roundup)
- Food Sensitivities
- Sugar
- Some drugs
- Infections, Parasites, Candida

If your animal has a leaky gut, that's where disease begins, so it is important to remove the factors listed above from their life. Read my chapter on autoimmune disease in my first book, **It Feels Good to Feel Good, Learn to Eliminate Toxins, Reduce Inflammation and Feel Great Again**. Leaky gut is a major factor in all chronic illnesses.

If your pet has itchy skin, irritable bowel syndrome, diarrhea, gas, or inflammatory bowel disease or if you suspect your pet has an allergy, then more than likely, your dog or cat has a food sensitivity or intolerance. One of the ways that food intolerances are born is that the same food is eaten repeatedly. Therefore, variety in the diet is important for your animal.

I took a sensitivity test, had 15 food sensitivities, and eliminating them from my diet was my first major step back to a pain-free life.

The same thing is true for cats and dogs. There is a company that tests for sensitivities. Food intolerance, or sensitivities, is the 3rd most common condition that causes your pets to suffer. And often, we are feeding our animals the same food over and over again. Fixing this is as easy, in most instances, of figuring out what the animal is sensitive to, and changing their food to avoid it and then adding variety.

Mind you; many conventional MDs do not believe in sensitivities, so they only test for allergies. Allergies are different. They are a very small percentage of foods that cause problems. Allergies could kill your pet. Sensitivities are, however, foods that cause a slow burn and cause inflammation over time. I don't know how Vets feel about sensitivities, but you need to be aware of this issue and have your pet tested if you think this could be a possibility. Once you know what the sensitivities are, it's a relatively easy fix. You change their food and avoid the items causing the intolerance.

I have found a company that does animal sensitivity testing.

"Developed by a world-renowned Veterinarian, Dr. Jean Dodds, NutriScan tests for the twenty-four most commonly ingested foods by dogs and cats to provide you with specific results as to your pet's food intolerances or sensitivities. Since it is a salivary test, you have the convenience to complete the test at home or your Veterinarian's Office. Best of all, you can have the results in approximately two weeks to help you put your companion animal on the right diet."[244]

The test is currently around $300, (in Feb 2020) but in my opinion, well worth the money it could save you at the Vets if you are shooting in the dark for a remedy for a sickly animal.

I recently received an email from HemoPet, which is Dr. Dodds organization. There is a new comprehensive testing for your pet.

"Decades of sustained experience in animal health research has taught us that CUSTOMIZED HEALTH NUTRITION is the key to sustaining the quality of life and prolonging the longevity of our companion pets.

"Knowledge is power, and The HemoPet Team wants to empower YOU! You can take control of your companion pets' health. You can allow them to live their very best lives for as long as possible. Our diagnostic tests, NUTRISCAN and CellBIO will provide you with the information allowing you to make the appropriate nutritional decisions for your companion. As an added BONUS we will include NutriGold, our "one-on-one" consultation to assure the ultimate benefits for your cherished pet companion.

"NutriScan, NutriGold and CellBIO profile $400

- "NutriScan Diagnostic Kit—Food Allergy Markers
- "CellBIO Markers Diagnostic Kit—Biomarkers for disease, cancer, obesity and inflammation

"Please visit us at nutriscan.org for updates—we would like your involvement."

Chapter 29

Vaccinations

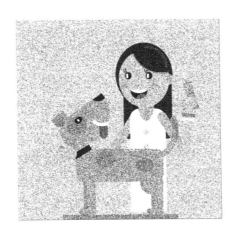
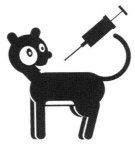

First, I want to note that I have never directly discussed vaccinations and children in either of my books. Vaccinations are a very complicated issue, and since you are the person that will deal with the consequences of whatever decision you make, I am not going to get in the middle of it. It is a personal decision. I have talked to moms who are vehement that their children should not be around an unvaccinated child and Moms who are vehement that they should be able to make their own decision. I have no doubt that there is over-vaccination taking place with our children, so my suggestion is that you research this subject thoroughly for your own family.[245]

I do know from what I have read that there is a small subset of children that are impacted negatively by some vaccinations. First get knowledgeable and then ask direct questions of your health care professionals.

When it comes to animals, there is also great concern about over vaccinations and the dangers that are involved in our pets. There are core vaccinations that must be given. I am quoting Dr. Karen Becker, a Holistic Vet, and Dr. Ronald Schultz, a leading researcher about animal vaccinations. Beyond these recommendations, if your Vet is recommending vaccinations beyond the "core" vaccinations, I suggest you get a second opinion and that you consult with a Holistic Vet.

These are the "core" vaccinations that Dr. Becker and Dr. Schultz recommend:

Distemper, parvo, and adenovirus (no parainfluenza) before 12 weeks old. Dr. Becker's tries to administer them around 9-10 weeks.

A second-round between 15-16 weeks. Two weeks after the second round, the dog is given a titer test. This ensures that the dog has been immunized and not just vaccinated. "An antibody titer is a measure of the concentration of antibodies in the blood, as determined by a test involving repeatedly diluting a blood sample and exposing those dilutions to an antigen. The shorthand is to refer to all measurements of antibody concentration as titers."[246]

Rabies is given at six months, and then it is required by law, a booster one year later and every three years after that.

The Goal Should Be to Immunize Pets, Not to Vaccinate Them Over and Over.[247]

Repeated boosters of core vaccines are not only unnecessary but also potentially dangerous to your pet's health.[248]

"**Titers, or quantitative antibody testing** can help determine your dog's protection from some diseases. Titer testing can be useful when a dog's vaccination history for distemper, adenovirus, and parvovirus is unknown—a positive result typically means he is considered protected.

"However, no test is 100% accurate, so in areas where these diseases run rampant, your Veterinarian may still recommend vaccinating. While titer testing for rabies is available, the law still requires that the dog be vaccinated since this is a fatal, zoonotic (i.e., can be spread to people) disease."

"The great news is Dr. John Robb has arranged for rabies, parvo, and distemper titer package for $55 (that you can submit yourself if your Vet doesn't do it)!"

Titer testing is also highly recommended to avoid over vaccinating your cats.[249]

If you do vaccinate your pet, ask your Holistic Veterinarian to provide a homeopathic vaccine detox such as Thuja (a common choice for all vaccines except rabies).

There are many other vaccinations that Vets will recommend every year. Again, do your research on this subject and get a second opinion and consult with a Holistic Vet.

These vaccinations are often in combination with other vaccinations that your pet may have had, and that are, therefore, unnecessary for your pet to get them again. Know what to ask. And ask to see the vial before any additional vaccinations are given by your Vet.

There is a lot of money to be made not only by over-vaccinating your pet but also from the wellness care you get when you go to the Vet this often. Wellness care is good, but over-vaccination can be harmful.

There is a long list of other vaccinations available. They may or may not be necessary depending upon your animal and the environment that you live in. Again, do your research and get a second opinion.

Also, important to note, most vaccinations come in one size for all. Whether your animal is very small or a 100 lb., behemoth, he gets the same shot. Question your Vet about this and the dangers involved.

Chapter 30

Steroids

PREDNISONE

One of the things that has been clarified in my mind as I have been researching about animals and medicine is that Conventional Vets are reactive, and Integrative Holistic Vets are proactive. Similarly, for humans, Conventional MD's are reactive, and Functional MD's and most Integrative MD's are proactive.[250]

If your dog or cat is suffering from a variety of conditions where your Conventional Vet wants to give your fur baby steroids, I suggest you get a second opinion from an Integrative Vet. You may be able to narrow down the "root cause" of the condition and save your animal the negative side effects of being put onto steroids.

"Why Steroid Therapy Can Be a Bad Idea"

DR. KAREN BECKER

"Two words: side effects.

"The biggest downside to steroids is they turn your pet's immune system off. When the immune system is shut down, your dog or cat will have a very hard time fighting secondary infections.

"Other side effects of steroid therapy can include:

- "Increased hunger and thirst
- "Increased urination
- "Lethargy
- "Gastrointestinal problems, including ulcers
- "Hair loss
- "A potbelly, which often signals the presence of Cushing's disease, a terrible condition that is known to result from steroid use
- "Blood clots
- "Diabetes
- "Pancreatitis
- "Secondary infections

"But my greatest concern about overuse of steroids is that the underlying condition causing your pet's symptoms, which is typically Inflammation, is usually left untreated."[251]

Steroids are reactionary. They only treat symptoms. I had a horrible reaction to steroids, so I would suggest that you do everything that you can to avoid giving them to your pet. (Or taking them yourself.) Now that I know what I do about human health, I would first make sure that the food that I am feeding my animal is "species-specific" and if it is not, that is the first thing I would do. I would run a CellBIO with Dr. Jean Dodds, which is a pre-clinical detection of chronic diseases in pets using saliva.

https://cellbiomarkers.org/order

I would run a sensitivity test that Dr. Jean Dodds has also devised to find out what items are causing sensitivities in my animal, which could be at the root of digestive disorders and leaky gut. This is the same way that I avoided steroids for my health.

I then healed my leaky gut.

LEAKY GUT

We have previously discussed what causes leaky gut (Chapter 28.)

Remember, as discussed in my chapter about your pet and the food you are feeding him, if your animal has a leaky gut, that's where disease begins, so it is important to remove the factors that cause leaky gut from their life. Read my chapter on autoimmune disease in my first book; **It Feels Good to Feel Good, Learn to Eliminate Toxins, Reduce Inflammation, and Feel Great Again**. Leaky gut is a major factor in all chronic illnesses.

As we discussed, if your pet has itchy skin, irritable bowel syndrome, diarrhea, gas, or inflammatory bowel disease or if you suspect your pet has an allergy, then more than likely, your dog or cat has a food sensitivity or intolerance. One of the ways that food intolerances are born is that the same food is eaten repeatedly. Therefore, variety in the diet is important for your animal. (Vets are taught in Vet school that changing an animal's food is not good for them. The opposite seems to be correct.)

I would take my pet to an Interactive Holistic Vet before I would let a Conventional Vet use steroids on my animal. While I was healing my pet's "leaky gut," I would use low toxin animal products. Keys Pure has a wonderful line of items that are low toxin for your pooch. They have a remarkable skin care system for dogs. https://www.keyspure.com/product-category/koda-dog/

To find an Integrative Holistic Veterinarian, you can go to https://www.ahvma.org

Again, I would do all of this before I would allow a Vet to administer steroids to my pet. The key, just like for humans, would be to figure out what is causing the condition in the first place. Steroids would be my last option, not my first.

There are times that you may want to use steroids, but I would let an Integrative Vet make that determination.

Chapter 31

Misc. other things you Should Know to Keep Your Pet Safe

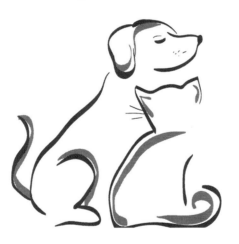

I encourage everyone to know where your local Emergency Veterinary clinic is and to have the number programmed into your phone. Also, post in on your refrigerator for fast use.

If you wouldn't eat it, don't feed it to your pet. You may choose to avoid raw meat, but you know which ones would not harm you.[252]

If the food is not on my good for snacks list, then do your research and make sure that what you are feeding your pet will not harm them.

If the food is on one list and not on the other, act with caution and don't feed it to cats or dogs. Or, do your research before you feed it to your pet.

Foods that are toxic to your dogs

Never feed them these:[253]

- Grapes
- Currants
- Raisins
- The seeds and pits of certain fruits—Peach pits, apricot seeds (kernels), plum pits, cherry pits, and apple seeds contain cyanide, which is truly a toxin.[254]
- Chocolate
- Caffeine
- Macadamia
- Mushrooms (some medicinal mushrooms can be helpful. Check with your Holistic Vet)
- Garlic and onion
- Potatoes
- Xylitol—This is in a lot of foods to make them sweet. This ingredient goes right through me. It can be lethal to your pet
- Gum
- Moldy foods
- Raw Seafood
- Liver (raw) only on an occasional basis
- Small, brittle bones
- Processed foods are not good for you, nor are they good for your pet. Fast food is also not good for your pet.

Foods that are toxic to your cats

Never feed them these:[255, 256, 257]

- Fat trimmings
- Raw meat
- Grapes
- Currants
- Raisins
- The seeds and pits of certain fruits—Peach pits, apricot seeds (kernels), plum pits, cherry pits, and apple seeds contain cyanide, which is truly a toxin.[258]
- Chocolate
- Macadamia
- Garlic and onion
- Xylitol—This is in a lot of foods to make them sweet. This ingredient goes right through me. It can be lethal to your pet
- Raw Eggs
- Alcohol
- Yeast Dough
- Raw Fish
- Green tomatoes
- Potatoes
- Milk products—Surprise, cats are lactose intolerant
- Caffeine
- Raw Seafood
- Liver (raw) only on an occasional basis
- Small, brittle bones
- Mustard seeds
- Tea (because it contains caffeine)
- Tomato leaves and stems (green parts)
- Walnuts
- Processed foods are not good for you, nor are they good for your pet. Fast food is also not good for your pet.

Toxic Plants

Some of these plants can be fatal if eaten. Always have the emergency phone number for the Emergency Vet in your area available and handy. Put it into your cell phone. Put it on your refrigerator.

There are different plants listed for cats and for dogs, but if the plant is on either list, I recommend that you do more research.

My suggestion is before you purchase any plants, especially indoor plants, do your research and make sure it is safe for your fur baby. I kept finding different lists, and I included what I found, but many of the plants on different lists vary from other lists, so be safe, and look up the plant before you purchase it and put your pet in danger. I always vote with caution. You many eliminate a house plant that wouldn't harm your pet, but no harm no foul.

Flowers, Bulbs, plants, and trees Poisonous to Dogs (There are indoor and outdoor plants on this list.)

- Autumn Crocus
- Begonia
- Chrysanthemum
- Daffodil
- Foxglove
- Larkspur
- Geranium
- Iris
- Autumn Crocus
- Azalea
- Caladium
- Cyclamen
- Kalanchoe
- Lilies are also very toxic to dogs
- Oleander
- Dieffenbachia

- Daffodils
- Lily of the Valley
- Sago Palm
- Tulips and Hyacinths—the bulbs are toxic, and the new growth in the spring is very toxic to dogs and cats
- Black Walnut—The tree itself isn't dangerous, but the nuts that fall to the ground can be. They start to decay very quickly and produce mold, so when a dog ingests them, they cause digestive upset and even seizures.
- Chinaberry
- Fruit trees
- Horse Chestnut (Buckeye)
- Japanese Yew
- Other nut trees: As a general rule, nuts aren't safe for dogs. Avoid letting your dog eat the nuts from almond, pecan, hickory, walnut, or other nut trees. Ingestion can cause gastrointestinal problems and intestinal blockage.
- Azalea and Rhododendron
- Holly
- Hydrangea
- Ivy
- Oleander
- Peony
- Sago Palm
- Any mushroom you cannot identify as safe
- Castor bean or castor oil plant (*Ricinus communis*)
- Cyclamen (*Cyclamen* spp.)
- Hemlock (Conium maculatum)
- English Ivy, both leaves and berries (*Hedera helix*)
- Mistletoe (*Viscum album*)
- Jade Plant
- Dracaena fragrans
- Golden Pothos
- Ficus Benjamina
- Flamingo Flower (Anthurium scherzerianum)

- Schefflera
- Amaryllis (Amaryllis sp.)
- A Philodendron
- Asparagus Fern (Asparagus setaceus)

Toxic around cats

- There are dangerous and benign lilies out there, and it's important to know the difference. Peace, Peruvian, and Calla lilies contain oxalate crystals that cause minor signs, such as tissue irritation to the mouth, tongue, pharynx, and esophagus—this results in minor drooling. The more dangerous, potentially fatal lilies are true lilies, and these include Tiger, Day, Asiatic, Easter, and Japanese Show lilies.
- Amaryllis (*Amaryllis* spp.)
- Autumn Crocus (Colchicum autumnale)
- Azaleas and Rhododendrons (*Rhododendron* spp.)
- Castor Bean (Ricinus communis)
- Chrysanthemum, Daisy, Mum (*Chrysanthemum* spp.)
- Cyclamen (*Cyclamen* spp.)
- Catnip (The ASPCA says that Catnip is toxic to cats. This is a new one on me)
- Daffodils, Narcissus (*Narcissus* spp.)
- Dieffenbachia (*Dieffenbachia* spp.)
- English Ivy (*Hedera helix*)
- Hyacinth (Hyacinthus orientalis)
- Kalanchoe (*Kalanchoe* spp.)
- Lily (*Lilium* sp.)
- Lily of the Valley (*Convallaria majalis*)
- Marijuana (Cannabis sativa)
- Oleander (Nerium oleander)
- Peace Lily (*Spathiphyllum* sp.)
- Pothos, Devil's Ivy (*Epipremnum aureum*)
- Sago Palm (Cycas revoluta)
- Spanish Thyme (Coleus ampoinicus)
- Tulip (*Tulipa* spp.)

- Yew (*Taxus* spp.)
- Jade Plant
- Dracaena fragrans
- Golden Pothos
- Ficus Benjamina
- Flamingo Flower (Anthurium scherzerianum)
- Schefflera
- Amaryllis (Amaryllis sp.)
- A Philodendron
- Asparagus Fern (Asparagus setaceus)

Fragrances that could impact your pets

Fragrances are usually toxic, whether they are in cosmetics, cleaning supplies, air fresheners, candles, etc. Even the things that are supposed to take "smells" out of the air of your home are toxic.

DO NOT USE any fragrance or non-fragrance sprays. They are harmful to your health. They are harmful to your pet. Beware of ingredients like natural fragrances. The word "natural" is not a legal term. Use my rule for buying products. If you don't know what it is, your body doesn't either, so pass and put it back on the shelf.

Always avoid fragrances for yourself and your pets.

I use essential oils now instead. When using essential oils, use a quality product. Otherwise, the oil might be synthetic, and therefore man-made and toxic—quality matters.

But Beware. Some essential oils are toxic to your pets

Here are the essential oils that are toxic to animals, so I wanted to post the list so that you take care of your fur babies. Avoid these essential oils if you have pets.

Some of these are from a recent blog post from Rocky Mountain oils,[259] which is the essential oil company that I use. Some of these are from previous research. There have been no studies on what oils are harmful to your pet to be around.

Never give them to your pet internally and watch your pet's reaction if you use any of these in the air. Your pet will let you know if it is something offensive to them. Always vote with caution. I used a flea product for pest control that had essential oils in it, and my cats were offended, so I never used it again.

Oils That May Be Toxic for Cats

- Bergamot
- Chamomile
- Cinnamon
- Clary Sage
- Eucalyptus
- Geranium
- Grapefruit
- Lavender
- Lemon
- Lemongrass
- Marjoram
- Orange
- Oregano
- Peppermint
- Pine
- Rose
- Rosemary
- Spearmint
- Tea Tree
- Wintergreen
- Ylang Ylang
- Cassia
- Citrus
- Clove
- Spruce
- Thyme

Cats have little bodies, so these are much more offensive for them than for a dog. If it is a problem for them, they will have a harder time processing the oil, and the impact on its body is greater. Always move forward with caution, and personally, I would avoid all the oils above on the list.

Oils That May Be Toxic for Dogs

- Chamomile
- Eucalyptus
- Geranium
- Grapefruit
- Orange
- Oregano
- Pine
- Tea Tree
- Wintergreen
- Clove
- Garlic
- Juniper
- Rosemary
- Thyme

This is the company that I use http://bit.ly/rockymtoils

More oils noted that could be toxic to your pets

Anise, birch, bitter almond, camphor, cassia, horseradish, hyssop, juniper, mugwort, mustard, oregano, pennyroyal, Ruta graveolens, sassafras, savory, tansy, thuja, wormwood, and yarrow.

Toxins in your home, cleaning supplies, laundry detergent, fabric softener

- Bleach
- Soap pods

- Most Detergents, I use Branch Basics (a one on the EWG scale) or Seventh Generation. EWG notes that most companies won't allow us to know the ingredients in their products. Don't buy them. Go to the EWG.com website look for a product's EWG rating or look for products from companies that practice transparency.
- Harsh chemical cleaners
- All fabric softeners, I use wool balls in my dryer
- Low chemical cleaners for your floors, I use Branch Basics
- White vinegar and then baking soda for toilets. My cats were always drinking water from the toilet, and I have seen a dog do that as well. You don't want them getting residual toxic chemicals.
- I use white vinegar to wipe down my kitchen counters, and then hydrogen peroxide as a chaser to clean my kitchen counters. I just read to leave the hydrogen peroxide on your counter for 10 minutes before wiping it off to kill all the germs and viruses. I soak my kitchen sponges in each solution every other day to kill germs and bacteria. Again 10 minutes each would kill everything you want to kill, but these are items safe for your skin to touch. These are safe for you and your pet.

Smoke

Smoke is very hard on your animal's bodies. "Living in a house with a smoker puts dogs, cats, and especially birds at greater risk of many health problems. Dogs exposed to second-hand smoke have more eye infections, allergies, and respiratory issues, including lung cancer."[260] Cats have issues with their lungs from second-hand smoke, but they also get mouth cancer from excessive grooming.

Test your home for mold.

It is as dangerous for your pets as it is for you.

Buy an air filter for each of the rooms where you spend a lot of time.

I suggest your living area or family room and your bedrooms.

Water quality

The water that comes out of your tap likely has toxic pollutants in it.

We put on an entire home system. At the very least, put a filter on your tap in the kitchen and use that water for your pet to drink. Make sure they get fresh water daily.

Mouse and rat poison

Keep these toxic chemicals in a cupboard high up where your sweet animal cannot get at them.

Prescriptions and Non-Prescription drugs

Keep your human drugs somewhere that your pet cannot get to them. Animals eating prescription and non-prescription drugs are the number one cause of animal poisoning.

Supplements and Holistic Solutions for your Pet

Wounds

Do not use Hydrogen Peroxide on your pet's wound. Do not use alcohol. If your pet has an open wound, the best thing you can do is wash it with filtered water. Then make a saline solution to help it heal.

There is a healing spray from a product line that is very low toxin, and they created it for their pet. The company is Keys Pure, and the product is Koda Omni Healing Spray.[261] They also make low toxin pet shampoos and face wash, and then they make a low toxin insect repellant. I love their products for humans, and when I first started using the line, I accidentally bought some dog products and used them on myself with great results. Woof, Woof. *smile*

Curcumin[262]

I am a huge believer in curcumin for my inflammation and pain. I no longer use any over the counter medications because they all are hard on either the gut or the liver. The same would be true for your pet since you do not want your pet to develop a leaky gut.

I am not surprised that Holistic Vets, like Dr. Becker[263] and Dr. Morgan[264], are also huge proponents of this for dogs and cats. Curcumin is the active ingredient in turmeric. I note two recipes for Golden Paste, which is a paste make from curcumin for your pet. I would use this in a heartbeat before a pharmaceutical. Remember to add a little black pepper because this makes the medicinal benefits bioavailable. Black pepper also has health benefits for your pet. I have noted a link to Dr. Becker's video about the benefits and her golden paste from a Vet's point of view.[265]

Ingredients[266]

> ½ cup organic powdered turmeric
> 1 cup filtered water
> 1/3 cup ethically sourced, organic coconut oil
> ½ - 1½ teaspoons freshly ground black pepper (increases bioavailability)
>
> Dosage typically ranges from ¼ teaspoon to 1 tablespoon daily, depending on the animal's size and the condition being treated. Pets who should not be given turmeric include those scheduled for surgery, those with gallbladder disease, diabetes, gastroesophageal reflux disease (GERD), hormone-sensitive tumors, and problems absorbing iron.
>
> The video for step by step how to make it
> https://bit.ly/animalgoldenpaste

This is Dr. Jody Morgan's recipe for golden paste:

Ingredients:

> 1 cup of warm water
> ½ cup of organic turmeric root powder
> 1/3 cup of organic coconut oil
> ½ tablespoon ground black pepper
> 1 tablespoon Ceylon cinnamon
>
> You can go to her website for a video as to how to make it.[267]
> They recommend that you freeze it in ice cube trays to keep it fresh for use.

Seasonal allergies—Use Quercetin

Give natural antihistamines—Dr. Becker also recommends quercetin, which is a bioflavonoid with anti-inflammatory, antioxidant, and antihistamine properties. I use quercetin for my own hay fever, and it works better for me than any antihistamine. It is known as "nature's Benadryl" because it's very effective at suppressing histamine release.

Dr. Becker says, "Bromelain and papain are proteolytic enzymes that increase absorption of quercetin, making it more effective. I like to combine bromelain and papain with vitamin C and quercetin because they have a great synergistic effect. Herbs such as stinging nettle, butterbur, sorrel, verbena, elderflower, and cat's claw have a documented history of helping animals combat seasonal allergic responses."

Buy Local Honey at your Farmers Market

Both John and I eat local honey to control our hay fever. I am not surprised that this also works well for pets.

Dr. Becker states: "Plant sterols and sterolins, which are anti-inflammatory agents, have also been used successfully to modulate the immune system toward a more balanced response in allergic patients. Locally produced honey contains a small amount of pollen from the local area that can help desensitize the body to local allergens over time." Usually, the best place to find local honey is at a farmer's market or neighborhood health food store. Check with your Veterinarian about the right dose for your dog or cat.

This is what commonly happens with seasonal environmental allergies. The more your pet is exposed to the allergens he's sensitive to, the more intense and long-lasting his allergic response becomes. That's why it's extremely important to begin addressing potential root causes at the first sign of an allergic response, no matter how mild it appears at its onset."

Vitamin D-3

Ask your Vet whether a D-3 supplement would benefit your pet.

Ubiquinol

Ubiquinol is often recommended for your pet companion's health, especially as your pet ages. It works at the Mitochondrial level in the cells of your pet's body.

Omega 3

This is very important to give as a supplement to your pet to enhance their health. Omega 3s are important for heart health, joint and bone health, it will help them avoid arthritis and improves movement throughout their lives, and it improves their skin and coat. Ask your Holistic Vet for their recommended brand. Fish oil Omega 3s are best, and Holistic Vets seem to prefer Krill Oil.

Enzymes

Although your pet makes these enzymes naturally, likely, they are not making enough to digest their food properly. Since you do not want your pet to get a "leaky gut," digestive enzymes are an important tool to keep your fur baby healthy.

Ask your Holistic Vet to recommend what brands to give to your pet.

These digestive enzymes include:

- Protease: Helps break down protein into amino acids
- Amylase: Helps break down carbohydrates
- Lipase: Helps with digesting fats
- Cellulase: For breaking down fiber

Prebiotics and Probiotics

Holistic Vets sell both, and both are important. Prebiotic feed the active probiotics in your animal's gut. And your animal needs healthy probiotics for his gut to remain healed and whole, and for his long-term health. Ask for recommendations from your Holistic Vet.

Things to discuss with your Holistic Vet

Before allowing your Vet to give a shot, get a list of ingredients and look them up. If the ingredients make you nervous, go to a Holistic Vet.

Ask if there are more natural ways to help your pet heal. Changing your fur baby's food? Healing his leaky gut? Always get options before you use pharmaceuticals. Remember, you must be your animal's advocate since they cannot talk for themselves.

And just like human health, our animal's health begins with quality food. **Food Quality Matters**. Your pet will live healthy and full lives if he/she is fed a species-specific healthy quality food.

Finally, practice gratitude that you have your lovely pet, and let them know how grateful you are that they are in your life. They will feel the energy, it will make your life sweeter that you shared your love with your companion animal, and it will make their life sweeter that you expressed it to them.

About the Author

Cheryl Meyer aka Cheryl M Health Muse

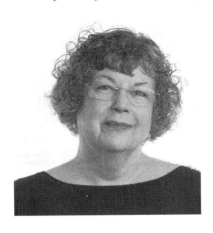

Cheryl is an entrepreneur and Type A personality. For the last 20 years, she has owned a sterling silver jewelry company where she designed jewelry for major retailers. Previously, she was a VP/General Store Manager for a major department store where she managed and coached over 200 employees to be their best.

Cheryl is as Integrative Nutrition Health Coach, aka Cheryl M Health Muse. She is a self-published author and an anti-toxin advocate.

Why did she become a health muse? To put it simply, Cheryl got sick, very sick. She had terrible pain from autoimmune disease and wasn't finding answers. She spent five years researching focusing on toxins in her life and ways to lower chronic stress. Having returned to relative wellness, she wants to share what she has learned to help you.

What can this health muse do for you? Cheryl will inspire you to take charge of your life and reduce your pain. She will help you find the answers you need for wellness. She wants her journey back to health to inspire you in your journey. Cheryl has a mission. She wants to help you to discover how to live clean and eat clean in a toxic world.

Cheryl is a newlywed (at a ripe old age) and married for five years to her perfect match in the greater Pasadena, California area. Together she and John have also now purchased a home in The Village of Oak Creek, Sedona, AZ, which they now spend half their time. Being in Sedona helps Cheryl slow down and find balance. John is the editor of her books and the producer of her TV shows and podcasts.

Cheryl happily reports, now in my 70's "I FEEL GREAT AGAIN, and so can you! I feel better than I did in my 50's."

Cheryl is available for individual and group coaching as well as public speaking and workshops. You can contact her at cherylnhealthmuse@gmail.com and follow her on Facebook as Cherylmhealthmuse. Join her private Facebook group, Feeling Good, Living Low Toxin.

Want to be the first to know? Follow what she is doing next and stay informed with the latest and the greatest new information. Her newsletters and blogs are all about living the good life pain-free without toxins and without deprivation and her tricks and tips to live low toxin and feel great. It's easy to join her mailing list from any page on her website which is also robust with great health information.

Watch her TV show on KGEM and KMAC community access TV in Monrovia, CA, Duarte, and Baldwin Park, CA. You can also watch the TV Episodes on her YouTube channel CherylMHealthMuse. You can find her books and shows on her new website heavenlytreepress.com, her publishing company website. She has her coaching and speaking website cherylmhealthmuse.com as well. Both offer valuable information to help you live your best, healthiest life.

Starting May 2020 watch for Cheryl's upcoming podcast, It Feels Good to Feel Good, Futureproof your Health and Tell Me Your Story, the Health Muse is In on RHG TV/Voice America. In the second part of her podcast, she will be interviewing others who have chronic illness and have also returned to wellness by making significant lifestyle changes. Cheryl wants to inspire you to do the same by listening to many success stories.

Her first book won 13 awards. It was revised and released as a second edition, Winter/Spring 2020. This is her second book, a blueprint for living low toxin in everyday life. She also has a Victory and Gratitude Journal available on Amazon. Cheryl has two more books planned in 2020, a pocketbook on Stress—3-minute stress exercises to release stress before it becomes chronic to improve daily productivity. She is also planning a cookbook, It Feels Good to Eat the Rainbow—recipes to cook with all the colors of fruits and vegetables for optimal health.

Nicholas Patton, Illustrator

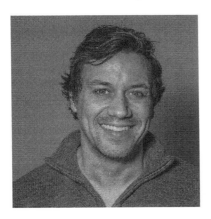

Nick Patton is a multidisciplinary artist living in Portland, OR. He received his BFA in illustration from Columbus College of Art and Design in Columbus, OH, and his MFA in Visual Studies from Pacific Northwest College of Art. Nick currently serves as the shop manager for PNCA's sculpture facilities while also completing freelance illustration projects and maintaining a fine art practice that ranges from printmaking to abstract sculpture.

For more information visit www.nickpattonart.com or contact Nick at nick_the_illustrator@yahoo.com

Special thanks to Nick for an outstanding job!!! Nick won two of the 13 awards that the first book won and was a total delight to work with.

Gizzy Dizzy, for additional illustrations, is an artist I found on Fiverr, and he stayed in my branding to provide wonderful additional illustrations for this book.

John Gins, Editor

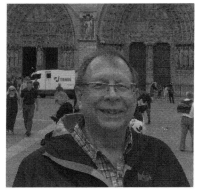

John is an officer of Heavenly Tree Press and CherylMhealthMuse.com. The mission of these companies is to help people be aware of the everyday toxins that we are all exposed to and what remedies can be taken to overcome exposure. John is the producer, editor, and technical support for the videos and books offered by Heavenly Tree Press. He provides Cheryl technical assistance for her on-line store.

His immediate interest is to help find ways to overcome the toxic lack of movement that has become prevalent in our society's sedentary lifestyle.

Before retiring in 2016, John worked in both applied statistics and computer technology for 43 years. In the Statistics arena, John wrote the prototype for CART in the '70s. This method for deriving decision trees from data is considered one of the earliest tools within the data mining community. Because of the computational demands of such automated statistical tools, John broadened his scope beyond statistics and consulting to computer systems and databases. John primarily consulted within the retail, financial, government, real estate, and internet industries. John is the primary author or significant contributor in over twenty publications.

John holds a BS in Mathematical Statistics from the University of Dayton and an MS in Mathematics from Wright State University in Dayton, Ohio.

John and Cheryl are ideal partners. They have been married now for five years.

Endnotes

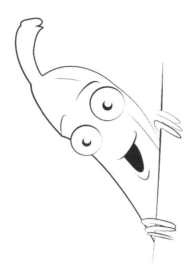

1 PREFACE

2   EWG https://www.ewg.org/research/body-burden-pollution-newborns

3 INTRODUCTION

4   https://www.amazon.com/Feels-Good-Feel-eliminate-inflammation/dp/0692827285

5 CHAPTER 1

6   https://www.youtube.com/watch?v=EVauROroe1Y

7 CHAPTER 2

8 https://www.tastend.com/

9 CHAPTER 3

10 If you haven't read my first book, you can buy it on my website cherylmhealthmuse.com or from Amazon

11 https://www.hindawi.com/journals/jnme/2019/2125070/

12 https://www.sciencebasedhealth.com/ContentPage.aspx?WebpageId=316

13 I did a class on Food Quality Matters and one of the classes was on color. The information listed in this article started with my interest in Dr. Deanna Minich's work and reading her books. She is all about color and her work inspired me to learn more and to incorporate her information into my own habits and teachings. The information in this chapter is Pulled from reading a variety of sources from

14 Dr. Deanna Minich

15 Dr. Josh Axe

16 Dr. David Jocker

17 Dr. Mark Hymen

18 Disabled World

19 Food Revolution Ocean Robbins

20 Food Matters website

21 Food for Life

22 Ohio State Your Plan for Health

23 I know that my body rejoices both mentally and physically when I incorporate all the colors of the rainbow into my diet. For more information, Start with reading Deanna Minich's work. The Rainbow Diet: A Holistic Approach to Radiant Health Through Foods and Supplements by Minich Ph.D. CNS, Deanna M. Conari Press; 1 edition | Jan 1, 2018 She is the authority that I follow on color.

24 Sehweiggert RM et al BR J Nutr. 2014 Feb. 111(3_ 490-8 doc 10,.1017/S9971114513992596

25 https://www.healthline.com/nutrition/leafy-green-vegetables

26 CHAPTER 4

27 It Feels Good to Feel Good, Learn to Eliminate Toxins, Reduce Inflammation and Feel Great Again. Available on Amazon or at https://cherylmhealthmuse.com/store/book/

28 It Feels Good to Feel Good, Learn to Eliminate Toxins, Reduce Inflammation and Feel Great Again. Available on Amazon or at https://cherylmhealthmuse.com/store/book/

29 This is a rating system used by Whole Foods that shows how humanely the animal was treated and how clean he was raised. A 4 or 5 chicken takes much longer to raise because growth hormones are not used to make the bird grow up and grow fat. In the end, he is still skinnier than the other birds.

30 I used to travel often to Thailand for my jewelry business and I couldn't get over how delicious their chickens were. Well, chickens back then, were mostly raised in backyards, and they would be comparable to a 4 or 5 chicken here today. They are worth it. We have forgotten how chicken raised without chemicals tastes.

31 As a root vegetable, potatoes absorb all of the pesticides, herbicides, and insecticides that are sprayed above the ground and then eventually make their way into the soil.

32 With potatoes, however, the chemical treatment is quite extensive.

33 During growing season— They get treated with fungicides

34 Before harvesting— They get sprayed with herbicides to kill off the fibrous vines

35 After being dug up— They get sprayed again to prevent them from sprouting

36 Quite often, the most important information about a food is what growers or "insiders" have to say about it.

37 Jeff Moyer, farm director at the Rodale Institute and former chair of the National Organic Standards Board, has been quoted as saying "I've talked with potato growers who say point-blank they would never eat the potatoes they sell. They have separate plots where they grow potatoes for themselves without all the chemicals."

38 https://livingmaxwell.com/health-risks-conventional-potatoes

39 USDA's Pesticide Data Program

40 It Feels Good to Feel Good, Learn to Eliminate Toxins, Reduce Inflammation and Feel Great Again. Available on Amazon or at https://cherylmhealthmuse.com/store/book/

41 https://julianbakery.com/product/pure-monk-sweetener/

42 CHAPTER 5

43 Food Matters http://store.foodmatters.com/?_ga=1.196868140.1893475740.1486086009

44 https://www.ncbi.nlm.nih.gov/pmc/articles/PMC3855594/

45 https://www.amazon.com/Melitta-640446-Pour-Over-Coffee-Brewer/dp/B0000CFLCT/ref=sr_1_1?keywords=melita+coffee+maker&qid=1569772893&s=books&sr=1-1-catcorr

46 I sell one in my Etsy and Woo stores, or you can buy one on Amazon.

47 https://therealfoodrds.com/tuscan-white-bean-dip/ Buy organic white beans in BPA free cans

48 https://www.thespruceeats.com/white-bean-hummus-dip-3377730 Buy organic white beans in BPA free cans

49 https://againstallgrain.com/2012/08/29/real-deal-chocolate-chip-cookies/ I buy

50 I buy Enjoy Life chocolate chips, soy free

51 https://nomnompaleo.com/post/38369819679/grain-free-dark-chocolate-cherry-scones

52 https://cherylmhealthmuse.com/2017/11/09/healthy-holiday-cooking-tips-crackers/

53 https://www.amazon.com/mayan-sweet-stevia-1027912539-Sachets/dp/B019EH98VQ/ref=sr_1_4?keywords=mayan+sweet+stevia+powder&qid=1569795172&s=gateway&sr=8-4

54 https://www.amazon.com/2-Quart-Bottles-Rectangular-Vintage-Storing/dp/B0799RGKW5/ref=sr_1_7?keywords=glass+1%2F2+gallon+bottles&qid=1569794842&s=books&sr=8-7

55 https://cynthiasass.com/sass-yourself/sass-yourself-blog/item/116-why-you-really-are-what-you-eat.html

56 CHAPTER 6

57 https://www.ams.usda.gov/local-food-directories/farmersmarkets

58 CHAPTER 7

59 It Feels Good to Feel Good, Learn to Eliminate Toxins, Reduce Inflammation and Feel Great Again available on my website or on Amazon.

60 I get these printed on heavy stock at Vista print. I put my picture on the card so that whoever I give it to remembers who I am to follow up with.

61 The Western pattern diet (WPD) or standard American diet (SAD) is a modern dietary pattern that is generally characterized by high intakes of red meat, processed meat, pre-packaged foods, butter, fried foods, high-fat dairy products, eggs, refined grains, potatoes, corn (and high-fructose corn syrup) and high-sugar drinks. The modern standard American diet was brought about by fundamental lifestyle changes following the Neolithic Revolution, and, later, the Industrial Revolution.

62 By contrast, a healthy diet has higher proportions of unprocessed fruits, nuts, vegetables, whole-grain foods, poultry, and fish. Wikipedia

63 https://perfectketo.com/canola-oil/

64 Picazzos

65 Tamaliza

66 Butterfly Burger

67 Lisa Dahl Restaurants in Sedona, Mariposa, Cucina Rustica, Dahl & Di Luca, Lisa Pisa, Butterfly Burger

68 ChocolaTree

69 The Enchantment Resort is out of town in Boynton Canyon, and it is spectacularly beautiful.

70 https://perfectketo.com/canola-oil/

71 Food Babe Restaurant Guide

72 Wikipedia

73 Lea Woodford

74 CHAPTER 8

75 Sautéed mushrooms roasted red and yellow bell peppers, sundried tomatoes, Applegate ham, Applegate Salami, Applegate Pepperoni, caramelized onions, different kinds of olives including kalamata, real cheese, vegan cheeses including Kite Hill ricotta, pineapple. Organic pizza sauce. And I make a white pizza sauce with soaked cashew nuts and seasonings.

76 https://giannamary.wordpress.com/ Her slogan is delicious, nutritious and nothing suspicious. Follow her blog for fantastic recipes and are just that.

77 CHAPTER 9

78 http://bit.ly/sittingaerobics I tried to find the Northwest video but it bit the dust back in the 90s. This is a 20-minute aerobic and resistance program that is very similar to what we used to do on the plane. Learn these and do some of them every 2 hours to circulate the blood in the body. You will feel so much better when it is time to exit the plane.

79 These pages also have excellent choices for airplane aerobics. Pick a series of these, get used to doing them at home, and then take the list of your favorites with you when you are travelling.

80 https://www.workingmother.com/11-quick-chair-exercises-that-work-as-well-as-going-to-gym#page-2

81 https://californiamobility.com/21-chair-exercises-for-seniors-visual-guide/

82 https://www.vivehealth.com/blogs/resources/chair-exercises-for-seniors

83 CHAPTER 10

84 Château du Clos Lucé is a relatively small 15th-century palace in the Loire town Amboise. The chateau was the childhood home of King Francis I but much more famously the palace where Leonardo da Vinci spent his final three years as the guest of the king of France.

85 CHAPTER 11

86 Chun Mok means Heavenly Tree

87 CHAPTER 12

88 It Feels Good to Feel Good, Learn to Eliminate Toxins, Reduce Inflammation and Feel Great Again. Available on my website at https://cherylmhealthmuse.com/book/ or at Amazon.

89 Dr. Mark Hyman Facebook post

90 http://bit.ly/salutethemorningcard

91 http://bit.ly/cameronmorningpages

92 http://bit.ly/weilsbreathing

93 I learned many of these exercises by doing yoga with Body and Brain Yoga. They have significantly lowered my stress. https://www.bodynbrain.com/

94 https://www.bellybuttonhealing.com

95 https://www.bellybuttonhealing.com

96 CHAPTER 13

97 Robert Emmons, perhaps the world's leading scientific expert on gratitude which he describes in a Greater Good essay, "Why Gratitude Is Good."

98 http://bit.ly/jacobsgratitudebook

99 CHAPTER 14

100 https://changeyourenergy.com/shop/609/belly-button-healing-kit

101 https://www.amazon.com/Feels-Good-Feel-eliminate-inflammation/dp/0692827285

102   CHAPTER 15

103   https://www.ewg.org/research

104   CHAPTER 16

105   https://thedyrt.com/magazine/lifestyle/self-care-tips/?fbclid=IwAR2Kx8dBhfaZE-KECprmLiDC_BKuh0IyB0U80G2tCiLOPxbYxesUnXjwhWvY

106   CHAPTER 17

107   https://en.wikipedia.org/wiki/Chatty_Cathy
108   https://business.wholelifechallenge.com/blog/creating-time-master-art-intentional-productivity/
109   https://www.amazon.com/Feels-Good-Feel-Celebrate-Gratitude/dp/173438591X/ref=sr_1_1?keywords=cheryl+meyer&qid=1579961956&sr=8-1

110   CHAPTER 18

111   http://www.mdcoalition.org/blog/self-care-connecting-with-nature
112   https://blog.thewellnessuniverse.com/healing-through-nature/

113   CHAPTER 19

114   https://www.mindbodygreen.com/articles/everything-you-need-to-know-about-forest-bathing
115   http://www.shinrin-yoku.org/shinrin-yoku.html
116   http://www.shinrin-yoku.org/shinrin-yoku.htm
117   https://www.mindbodygreen.com/articles/why-national-parks-should-be-a-part-of-our-public-health-strategy
118   http://www.shinrin-yoku.org/shinrin-yoku.html
119   https://www.mindbodygreen.com/articles/everything-you-need-to-know-about-forest-bathing
120   https://www.mindbodygreen.com/articles/why-national-parks-should-be-a-part-of-our-public-health-strategy
121   https://www.ilchi.com/breathe-with-the-trees/
122   https://www.ilchi.com/breathe-with-the-trees/

123 https://www.mindbodygreen.com/0-20793/10-great-reasons-to-get-outside-more-often.html

124 https://www.dailymail.co.uk/sciencetech/article-5653667/The-heartbeat-tree-Scientists-discover-plants-pulsate-night.html

125 https://returntonow.net/2018/04/29/trees-have-a-heartbeat-scientists-discover/

126 https://thedyrt.com/magazine/lifestyle/self-care-tips/?fbclid=IwAR2Kx8dBhfaZEKE-CprmLiDC_BKuh0IyB0U80G2tCiLOPxbYxesUnXjwhWvY

127 https://www.growwilduk.com/blog/5-simple-steps-practising-shinrin-yoku-forest-bathing

128 https://www.growwilduk.com/blog/5-simple-steps-practising-shinrin-yoku-forest-bathing

129 https://www.drperlmutter.com/on-the-healing-power-of-nature/

130 https://www.mindbodygreen.com/articles/everything-you-need-to-know-about-forest-bathing

131 https://www.mindbodygreen.com/articles/the-science-of-forest-bathing

132 https://www.mindbodygreen.com/articles/the-science-of-forest-bathing

133 https://www.mindbodygreen.com/articles/the-science-of-forest-bathing

134 https://www.mindbodygreen.com/articles/the-science-of-forest-bathing

135 https://www.mindbodygreen.com/articles/the-science-of-forest-bathing

136 https://www.mindbodygreen.com/articles/the-science-of-forest-bathing

137 https://www.mindbodygreen.com/0-25512/the-magic-of-forest-bathing-how-to-incorporate-it-into-your-selfcare-routine.html

138   CHAPTER 20

139 Mosquitomagnet.com

140 https://www.treehugger.com/health/7-reason-mosquitoes-bite-some-people-more-others.html I used their 7 points but rewrote them from my point of view.

141 Not her real name, I am protecting her identity.

142 https://www.ewg.org/research/ewgs-guide-bug-repellents-age-zika/what-you-can-do-about-zika

143 https://www.absorbentproductsltd.com/does-diatomaceous-earth-kill-ants/

144 COMMON BUGS Earth Friendly Ways to Control Them (Pesticides are Weapons of Mass Destruction)

145 COMMON BUGS Earth Friendly Ways to Control Them (Pesticides are Weapons of Mass Destruction)

146 COMMON BUGS Earth Friendly Ways to Control Them (Pesticides are Weapons of Mass Destruction)

147 COMMON BUGS Earth Friendly Ways to Control Them (Pesticides are Weapons of Mass Destruction)

148 COMMON BUGS Earth Friendly Ways to Control Them (Pesticides are Weapons of Mass Destruction)

149 http://bit.ly/pantrymothtraps

150 COMMON BUGS Earth Friendly Ways to Control Them (Pesticides are Weapons of Mass Destruction)

151 COMMON BUGS Earth Friendly Ways to Control Them (Pesticides are Weapons of Mass Destruction)

152 COMMON BUGS Earth Friendly Ways to Control Them (Pesticides are Weapons of Mass Destruction)

153 COMMON BUGS Earth Friendly Ways to Control Them (Pesticides are Weapons of Mass Destruction)

154   CHAPTER 21

155 https://www.helpguide.org/articles/healthy-eating/healthy-food-for-kids.htm

156 EWG https://www.ewg.org/research/body-burden-pollution-newborns

157 EWG https://www.ewg.org/research/body-burden-pollution-newborns

158 https://paleoleap.com/how-a-fathers-diet-affect-his-babys-health/

159 https://livehealthybewell.com/podcast/multi-generational-health-damage/

160 https://www.livescience.com/45681-vaginal-birth-vs-c-section.html

161 https://www.healthline.com/health-news/should-babies-born-via-c-section-get-microbial-seeding#How-can-this-help?

162 https://www.healthline.com/health-news/should-babies-born-via-c-section-get-microbial-seeding

163 https://www.webmd.com/parenting/baby/nursing-basics#1

164 https://www.healthychildren.org/English/ages-stages/baby/breastfeeding/Pages/Why-Breastfeed.aspx

165 https://www.healthline.com/health-news/should-babies-born-via-c-section-get-microbial-seeding#The-risks-of-seeding

166 https://www.parents.com/baby/breastfeeding/basics/the-benefits-of-breastfeeding/

167 https://www.parents.com/baby/breastfeeding/basics/the-benefits-of-breastfeeding/

168 https://www.parents.com/baby/breastfeeding/basics/the-benefits-of-breastfeeding/

169 https://www.medela.com/breastfeeding/mums-journey/breastfeeding-benefits-baby

170 Some mothers are physically unable to breast feed.

171 https://wellnessmama.com/53999/baby-formula-options/

172 If you don't know what it means to be GMO, I have a chapter about organic, conventional and GMO in my first book, It Feels Good to Feel Good, Learn to Eliminate Toxins, Reduce Inflammation and Feel Great Again.

173 http://beetrootbrooke.com/blog/2018/2/nourishingnext

174 Pottery Barn carried silicone elephants, cats and dog bowls and mats.

175 https://www.instagram.com/unicornsuperfoods/

176 https://www.instagram.com/nutritiouslydelicious_/

177 http://beetrootbrooke.com/blog/2018/2/nourishingnext

178 http://drhyman.com/blog/2014/03/06/top-10-big-ideas-detox-sugar

179 https://sietefoods.com/

180 https://www.tastend.com/

181   **CHAPTER 22**

182 https://www.velux.com/indoorgeneration

183 https://qz.com/quartzy/1480959/if-you-love-nature-here-are-20-words-to-say-aloud/

184 https://www.amazon.com/gp/product/1487005385/ref=ppx_yo_dt_b_asin_title_o00_s00?ie=UTF8&psc=1

185 https://www.mindbodygreen.com/articles/the-science-behind-why-nature-is-so-restorative

186 https://www.mindbodygreen.com/articles/why-you-want-to-raise-wild-child

187 https://www.mindbodygreen.com/articles/why-you-want-to-raise-wild-child

188 https://www.washingtonpost.com/news/parenting/wp/2018/05/30/kids-dont-spend-nearly-enough-time-outside-heres-how-and-why-to-change-that/

189 http://nwf.org/greenhour.

190 http://nwf.org/greenhour.

191 https://childmind.org/article/ideas-for-getting-your-kids-into-nature/

192   CHAPTER 23

193 https://www.consumerreports.org/consumerist/10281160/

194 https://www.washingtonpost.com/news/wonk/wp/2017/06/15/seven-percent-of-americans-think-chocolate-milk-comes-from-brown-cows-and-thats-not-even-the-scary-part/

195 https://www.consumerreports.org/consumerist/10281160/

196 https://www.consumerreports.org/consumerist/10281160/

197 https://www.consumerreports.org/consumerist/10281160/

198 https://www.washingtonpost.com/news/wonk/wp/2017/06/15/seven-percent-of-americans-think-chocolate-milk-comes-from-brown-cows-and-thats-not-even-the-scary-part/

199 https://www.express.co.uk/life-style/food/712737/avocados-come-from-animals-Kids-shocking-lack-of-food-knowledge-exposed

200 Kitchen Literacy: How We Lost Knowledge of Where Food Comes from and Why We Need to Get It Back 2nd ed. Edition by Ann Vileisis Island Press; 2nd ed. edition (March 15, 2010)

201 https://www.alternet.org/2008/05/how_we_lost_knowledge_of_where_food_comes_from_and_why_we_need_to_get_it_back/

202 https://indianapublicmedia.org/eartheats/five-reasons-care-food-comes-from.php

203 https://indianapublicmedia.org/eartheats/five-reasons-care-food-comes-from.php

204 https://www.thespruce.com/container-garden-projects-kids-will-love-847955

205 https://kidsgardening.org/garden-activities-throw-a-garden-birthday-party/

206 https://kidsgardening.org/garden-activities-throw-a-garden-birthday-party/

207 http://bit.ly/kidsgardeninggloves

208 http://bit.ly/smallwheelbarrow

209 http://bit.ly/tinyredwagons

210 http://bit.ly/babytoywateringcan

211 http://bit.ly/ladybugwateringcan

212 https://www.diyncrafts.com/4732/repurpose/25-foods-can-re-grow-kitchen-scraps

213 http://bit.ly/hometowergarden

214   CHAPTER 24

215 https://psychologia.co/types-of-thinking/

216 https://medium.com/the-mission/the-importance-of-reading-fiction-7f57546a229b

217 https://medium.com/the-mission/the-importance-of-reading-fiction-7f57546a229b

218 Ann Patchett

219 https://medium.com/the-mission/the-importance-of-reading-fiction-7f57546a229b

220 https://www.greenchildmagazine.com/reading-to-unborn-baby/

221 https://childcarelounge.com/pages/the-importance-of-reading-aloud-to-children

222 An Australian educator and writer of popular children's books

223 https://childcarelounge.com/pages/the-importance-of-reading-aloud-to-children

224 https://www.pbs.org/parents/thrive/why-reading-aloud-to-kids-helps-them-thrive

225 http://theconversation.com/read-aloud-to-your-children-to-boost-their-vocabulary-111427

226 https://www.pbs.org/parents/thrive/why-reading-aloud-to-kids-helps-them-thrive

227 https://www.pbs.org/parents/thrive/why-reading-aloud-to-kids-helps-them-thrive

228 https://theconversation.com/research-shows-the-importance-of-parents-reading-with-children-even-after-children-can-read-82756

229 https://www.pre-kpages.com/reading-aloud-to-kids/

230 https://www.pre-kpages.com/reading-aloud-to-kids/

231 https://theconversation.com/dinnertime-storytelling-makes-kids-voracious-readers-47318

232 https://theconversation.com/dinnertime-storytelling-makes-kids-voracious-readers-47318

233 https://www.pbs.org/parents/learn-grow/age-8/literacy/reading

234 https://www.washingtonpost.com/news/parenting/wp/2017/02/16/why-its-important-to-read-aloud-with-your-kids-and-how-to-make-it-count/

235   CHAPTER 25

236 https://www.healthychildren.org/English/safety-prevention/at-play/Pages/Swimming-Pool-Safety.aspx

237 https://guardianpoolfence.com/5-tips-swimming-pool-safety-children/

238 https://kidshealth.org/en/parents/water-safety-pools.html

239 https://www.webmd.com/children/features/new-pool-safety-gadgets-help-prevent-drowning#2

240   CHAPTER 26

241 The Truth About Pet Cancer, and documentary released in 2017.

242 The Truth About Pet Cancer, and documentary released in 2017

243 The Truth About Pet Cancer, and documentary released in 2017

244 The Truth About Pet Cancer, and documentary released in 2017 Karen Becker

245 The Truth About Pet Cancer, and documentary released in 2017.

246   CHAPTER 27

247   Dr. Mark Hyman

248 TTAC

249 Read all about Glyphosate (Round Up) in It Feels Good to Feel Good, Learn to Eliminate Toxins, Reduce Inflammation and Feel Great Again, my first book.

250 Michelle Jeongin Moon, Gut Health Workshop, February 2020, Body and Brain, Pasadena, CA

251 https://www.healthline.com/nutrition/synthetic-vs-natural-nutrients#section5

252 https://truthaboutpetfood.com/new-to-the-truth/

253 TTAC

254 https://www.medicalnewstoday.com/articles/320156#Sucrose-and-cancer-today

255 https://healthypets.mercola.com/sites/healthypets/archive/2020/02/08/clean-label-pet-food.aspx?cid_source=petsnl&cid_medium=email&cid_content=art1H-L&cid=20200208Z1&et_cid=DM450873&et_rid=806371787

256 https://www.cornucopia.org/2015/11/new-report-exposes-dangerousun-healthy-pet-food/

257 Karen Becker Blog https://healthypets.mercola.com/sites/healthypets/archive/2020/02/08/clean-label-pet-food.aspx?cid_source=petsnl&cid_medium=e-mail&cid_content=art1HL&cid=20200208Z1&et_cid=DM450873&et_rid=806371787

258 https://truthaboutpetfood.com/new-study-suggests-rice-in-pet-food-can-lead-to-chronic-arsenic-exposure/

259 https://www.cornucopia.org/2015/12/the-truth-about-pet-food/

260 https://www.cornucopia.org/2015/12/the-truth-about-pet-food/

261 https://www.scientificamerican.com/article/the-carrageenan-controversy/

262 https://feline-nutrition.org/health/feline-inflammatory-bowel-disease-nature-and-treatment

263   CHAPTER 28

264 https://healthypets.mercola.com/sites/healthypets/archive/2015/11/08/best-to-worst-pet-food-types.aspx?x_cid=youtube

265 https://healthypets.mercola.com/sites/healthypets/archive/2015/11/08/best-to-worst-pet-food-types.aspx?x_cid=youtube

266 https://healthypets.mercola.com/sites/healthypets/archive/2015/11/08/best-to-worst-pet-food-types.aspx?x_cid=youtube

267 https://healthypets.mercola.com/sites/healthypets/archive/2015/11/08/best-to-worst-pet-food-types.aspx?x_cid=youtube

268 https://healthypets.mercola.com/sites/healthypets/archive/2015/11/08/best-to-worst-pet-food-types.aspx?x_cid=youtube

269 https://healthypets.mercola.com/sites/healthypets/archive/2015/11/08/best-to-worst-pet-food-types.aspx?x_cid=youtube

270 https://healthypets.mercola.com/sites/healthypets/archive/2015/11/08/best-to-worst-pet-food-types.aspx?x_cid=youtube

271 https://healthypets.mercola.com/sites/healthypets/archive/2015/11/08/best-to-worst-pet-food-types.aspx?x_cid=youtube

272 https://www.hemopet.org/hemolife-diagnostics/dog-and-cat-nutriscan/

273   CHAPTER 29

274 https://www.avma.org/javma-news/2016-07-01/titer-or-revaccinate

275 https://healthypets.mercola.com/sites/healthypets/archive/2019/05/18/over-vaccinating-pets.aspx

276 https://www.youtube.com/watch?v=ETpOIriQ4Tc

277 https://animalwellnessmagazine.com/titer-testing-cats/

278   CHAPTER 30

279 https://healthypets.mercola.com/sites/healthypets/archive/2010/08/17/stop-using-pet-steroids-until-you-read-these-disturbing-truths.aspx

280   CHAPTER 31

281 https://www.hemopet.org/toxic-foods-for-dogs-are-they-truly-toxic-part-1/?utm_source=Clients&utm_campaign=1237dd63e3-EMAIL_

CAMPAIGN_2020_02_17_02_58&utm_medium=email&utm_term=0_2a-b0e3771c-1237dd63e3-234813685

282 https://www.hemopet.org/toxic-foods-for-dogs-are-they-truly-tox-ic-part-1/?utm_source=Clients&utm_campaign=1237dd63e3-EMAIL_CAMPAIGN_2020_02_17_02_58&utm_medium=email&utm_term=0_2a-b0e3771c-1237dd63e3-234813685

283 https://www.preventivevet.com/cats/human-foods-you-should-not-give-to-your-cat

284 https://www.homeoanimal.com/blogs/blog-pet-health/toxic-foods-for-cats

285 https://www.homeoanimal.com/blogs/blog-pet-health/toxic-foods-for-cats

286 https://www.hemopet.org/toxic-foods-for-dogs-are-they-truly-tox-ic-part-1/?utm_source=Clients&utm_campaign=1237dd63e3-EMAIL_CAMPAIGN_2020_02_17_02_58&utm_medium=email&utm_term=0_2a-b0e3771c-1237dd63e3-234813685

287 https://www.rockymountainoils.com/learn/are-essential-oils-safe-for-pets/?rs_oid_rd=3029519607433380&utm_source=Email&utm_medium=RetSci&utm_campaign=ProductHighlight202002_Pets&utm_term=Email-RetSci-ProductHighlight202002_Pets-Info_Button-20200220&utm_content=Info_Button

288 https://vcahospitals.com/know-your-pet/the-effects-of-second-hand-smoke-on-pets

289 https://www.keyspure.com/product/koda-omnicare-spray/

290 https://healthypets.mercola.com/sites/healthypets/videos.aspx

291 https://healthypets.mercola.com/sites/healthypets/dr-karen-becker.aspx

292 https://drjudymorgan.com/

293 https://www.facebook.com/doctor.karen.becker/videos/10153928990512748/

294 https://healthypets.mercola.com/sites/healthypets/archive/2019/11/22/turmer-ic-benefits-for-pets.aspx

295 https://drjudymorgan.com/blogs/recipes/how-to-make-golden-paste

Made in the USA
San Bernardino, CA
28 June 2020